Good Stress, Bad Stress

Also by Barry Lenson

Simple Steps
(WITH DR. ARTHUR CALIANDRO)

Take Control of Your Life
(WITH DR. RICHARD SHOUP)

Multicultural and Ethnic Marketing
(WITH ALFRED L. SCHRIEBER)

BARRY LENSON

Good Stress, Bad Stress

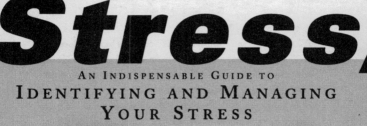

An Indispensable Guide to
Identifying and Managing
Your Stress

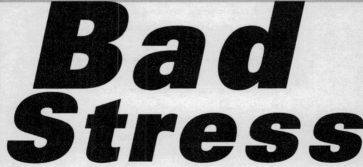

MARLOWE & COMPANY
NEW YORK

GOOD STRESS, BAD STRESS:
An Indispensable Guide to Identifying and Managing Your Stress
Copyright © 2002 by Barry Lenson

Published by
Marlowe & Company
An Imprint of Avalon Publishing Group Incorporated
161 William Street, 16th Floor
New York, NY 10038

Library of Congress Cataloging-in-Publication Data
Lenson, Barry.
Good stress, bad stress / Barry Lenson.
p. cm.
ISBN 1-56924-529-0 (trade paper)
1. Stress (Psychology) 2. Stress management. I. Title.
BF575.S75 .L36 2002
155.9'042—dc21   2002019878

9 8 7 6 5 4 3 2 1

Designed by Pauline Neuwirth, Neuwirth & Associates, Inc

Printed in the United States of America
Distributed by Publishers Group West

For Fran and Olivia,
who chase away
the bad stress and
make my life a joy

Contents

PART III:
Minimizing the Damage that Bad Stress Is Causing in Your Life

PREFACE

Fifty years ago, virtually no one used the word "stress" to describe personal anxiety. In the decades since then, stress has become the most pervasive psychological complaint in our society and a contender for the most widespread health problem of any kind.

How pervasive is stress? Consider these statistics, compiled by the American Psychological Association:

- 75 to 90 percent of all physician office visits in the United States are for stress-related complaints.
- 43 percent of all American adults suffer some kind of adverse health effects from stress.
- Stress costs American business more than $300 billion each year (about $7,500 per employee) due to absenteeism, reduced productivity, and health benefits paid.

Or these statistics, which tell us that 2001 is a contender for the most stressful year in history:

- A month after the World Trade Center attacks in September 2001, national polls determined that between 60 and 80 percent of all Americans were suffering from some degree of posttraumatic stress disorder.

▶ In October 2001, the Gallup Organization reported that 36 percent of all Americans felt "worried" about events in the world. One month later that percentage surged to 45.

Are You Stressed?

Those are troubling statistics. But they don't touch on the worst part of the story: the damage stress can do to *your* life.

Left unchecked, stress has the potential to destabilize your loving relationships, rob the joy from your family life, and damage your most important friendships. It can render your working life unpleasant or even impossible.

And we all know that stress can make you sick, sometimes *very* sick, by increasing the likelihood that you will suffer a stroke, heart disease, hypertension, ulcers, colitis, or other serious physical ailments.

In short, if stress is left unchecked, it can render life's routines difficult, unpleasant, and sometimes excruciating. It might even shorten your life.

Good Stress

Yet did you know that there is such a thing as *good stress*? The concept comes as a surprise to many people until they stop to recall how often stress actually exerted a beneficial influence on their lives.

I have benefitted from stress and you might have too.

Better performance. Your nervousness before an important event was unpleasant, yet it spurred you to perform at a very high level. You might have been preparing an important presentation at work, doing your warmups before a crucial game with your softball team, driving to a critical meeting you were about to lead at city hall, or setting up the tables before an important dinner you had to host. You felt the tension, you were wound up tight, but your stress helped you reach unexpected levels of accomplishment.

A sense of flow. Your stress melded imperceptibly into something you did not expect: a state of flow. While you were under pressure to complete an important project at work, something shifted and the task seemed to "finish itself." Or perhaps all your pre-performance nerves seemed to disappear before you stepped onto the stage to perform your part in a play. Suddenly you seemed to be not an actor on the stage but actually one of the characters in the drama. At times we have all felt this wonderful sensation called *flow*. Professional athletes call it "being in the zone," and if you have been there, you know how effortless it feels. You might not have stopped to realize that flow is a gift of positive stress.

Unexpected progress and accomplishment. You attacked a difficult or unpleasant task head-on and experienced a sudden surge of positive emotions afterward. It might have been a dreaded confrontation with your boss or a ticklish conversation with your spouse about family finances. But with the event behind you, you sensed that new possibilities had suddenly opened before you and you felt great. That's good stress masquerading as bad. All it takes is the right kind of action from you to unlock its benefits.

So we see that not all stress is bad. Good stress has helped me do things better, achieve more, and bring joy to the process of living. If you stop to consider your own life, I believe you will discover that good stress has helped you too.

Without good stress, you and I could never move to a higher plane of accomplishment and joy that can make us and our lives exceptional. We would never tell another person, "I want to share my life with you." We would never become parents. We would never appear in plays, perform music, or make speeches. We would never learn to ride bicycles, swim, run marathons, or earn black belts. We would never apply for challenging jobs, start our own companies, make deals, or pursue our most cherished dreams. I could never have written this book without a healthy dose of good stress delivered in the form of deadlines, high expectations from the publisher, and self-discipline.

You and I are not alone in the knowledge that stress can be not only good but an essential part of a fulfilling life that lifts us to a new level of accomplishment and happiness. As we will discover in the pages ahead, researchers are discovering more and more about the difference between good stress and bad. They are finding new ways to turn stress from an enemy into a friend.

What This Book Will Do for You

Good Stress, Bad Stress offers a simple, highly effective approach for reducing the damage done by bad stress and increasing the benefits you receive from good stress.

First, you will find out about exciting research findings that show conclusively that there are two kinds of stress: *good* and bad. After taking the Personal Stress Inventory, a unique self-administered test, you will have a comprehensive blueprint of the many areas where stress is at work in your life. You will then learn some remarkably effective ways to determine which of those life stresses are good, and which are bad. You are now ready to begin processing your life stress using the highly effective new techniques unique to *Good Stress, Bad Stress.*

Second, you will begin to enjoy the many benefits that good stress can offer you. Sometimes it will be immediately apparent which of your life stresses are good, and which are bad. At other times, you won't understand the true nature of one of your stresses until you take action on it. (Often, stresses we believe to be bad turn out to be good when we take action on them.) In either case, you will discover the remarkable benefits that follow the realization that *not all stress is bad.*

Third, you will apply effective ways to minimize the negative impact of bad stress in your life in areas where it *cannot* be changed to good. Because not all bad stresses in our lives can be made to go away quickly. Consider chronic health conditions, troubled relationships with children, challenges of ailing parents, and the career impasses that take time to resolve. Such problems tend to linger. Yet the good news is, there are many effective techniques to minimize the damaging effects that these negative stressors can have. Despite bad stresses, our lives can be kept in healthy balance and made worth living.

This is the groundbreaking new stress-fighting program you will discover in *Good Stress, Bad Stress.*

PART I:

Discovering the Good and Bad Stresses in Your Life

Which of the stresses in your life are good? Which are bad?

Let's take a closer look at both kinds of stress and gain a new understanding into how stress might be impacting on your life.

1

IS STRESS GOOD OR BAD?

On July 25, 2001, a provocative article, "Learning How to Work with the Good Stress, Live Without the Bad," appeared in *The Wall Street Journal*. Written by reporter Sue Shellenbarger, it presented recent findings in answer to a question that had been the subject of scientific research for half a century: Could it be that some types of stress actually produce positive outcomes in our lives, do no physical damage to us, and make us happier and healthier?

"Arguably," Shellenbarger concluded, "good stress is the kind that motivates and excites, the kind most likely to yield good results on the job. Bad stress is the kind that fouls performance."

In other words, there is such a thing as "good" stress, a little-recognized counterpart to the negative stress most of us deal with every day.

That news struck many readers as surprising and possibly revolutionary. Yet before we take a close look at the research Shellenbarger was reporting, let's take a moment to get a better understanding of what stress is all about.

Hans Selye: Father of Modern Stress

"Stress" is a word used so often today in our society, it's easy to assume that it has always been part of our working vocabulary. Not so.

It's true that Sigmund Freud dealt with stress in many writings, including *The Problem of Anxiety*. So did the Swiss psychologist Carl Jung in *The Undiscovered Self* and other works. Yet neither of these giants gave particular notice to stress per se or singled it out for special study.

The psychologist who first recognized stress (the "father" of modern stress, if you will) was Hans Selye, a scientist who gave birth to the concept of stress in his book *The Stress of Life*, published in 1956. Yet even in that book, Selye did not dwell extensively on the *psychological* aspects of stress.

The Stress of Life reports that when Selye was a medical student at the University of Prague in 1925, he noticed that most people when becoming ill developed an assortment of symptoms that included aches and pains, a coated tongue, and a loss of appetite. Because similar symptoms preceded many different diseases, he believed he had identified a specific pre-disease *stress syndrome* that could be analyzed apart from the ailment that followed.

Through years of laboratory experiments, Selye pursued the possibility that stress is the body's attempt to establish equilibrium in reaction to negative stimuli from outside, especially the onset of disease. By the time he published his revised edition of *The Stress of Life* in 1976, Dr. Selye had spent a half-century studying the effects of stress on both humans and upon the brains and internal organs of laboratory animals. He announced his beliefs that there are actually two kinds of stress: bad and good.

He called them *eustress* and *distress*. As Selye wrote:

> We must, however, differentiate within the general concept of stress between the unpleasant or harmful variety, called "distress" (from the Latin dis = bad, as in dissonance, disagreement) and "eustress" (from the Greek eu = good, as in euphonia, euphoria). During both eustress and distress the body undergoes virtually the same nonspecific responses to the various positive or negative stimuli act-

**ing upon it. However, the fact that eustress causes much
less damage than distress graphically demonstrates that it
is "how you take it" that determines, ultimately, whether
one can adapt successfully to change.**

Why didn't Dr. Selye's revolutionary belief that stress could be
either good or bad attract more widespread attention? Surely
Selye had tried to let people know. He had even published a book,
Stress Without Distress, in 1974, where he made this remarkable
testament to the power of stress to make our lives better:

> **Stress is the spice of life. Since stress is associated with
> all types of activity, we could avoid most of it only by
> never doing anything. Who would enjoy a life of no runs,
> no hits, no errors? Besides . . . certain types of activities
> have a curative effect and actually help to keep the stress
> mechanism in good shape.**

Stress Becomes a Mainstream Concern

As Selye pursued his stress studies, the topic was quickly taken
up by many other researchers. Mortimer H. Appley and
Richard Trumbull wrote a pioneering article, "On the Concept
of Psychological Stress," which appeared in *Psychological Stress:
Issues in Research*, in 1967. Another trailblazer was Richard S.
Lazarus, who wrote the book *Cognitive and Coping Processes in
Emotion*, in 1974. A growing number of books, articles, and
specialized periodicals appeared on the topic of stress.

Suddenly stress became mainstream. Transcendental Meditation, a maharishi's system of mantra-based, anxiety-reducing
meditation, gained widespread acceptance on college campuses
in the 1960s and 1970s. The technique even appeared in
westernized garb in Herbert Benson's 1975 bestseller *The
Relaxation Response*, a self-primer on meditation that remains
popular today.

Depictions of Stress in Art

As is often the case, artists and writers were well ahead of scientists. What is Kafka's *Metamorphosis*, the tale of a man who wakes up in bed one morning to discover that he has become a giant beetle, if not a tale propelled by stress? Or what about Robert Schumann's four disquieting symphonies, written a century earlier by a man whose life was so troubled, he finally jumped off a bridge to still the sounds he heard in his head? And let's not forget expressionist paintings, especially Edvard Munch's famous *The Scream*, painted back in 1893. There are few clearer depictions of what it feels like to be hopelessly mired in stress.

Then there is W. H. Auden's 1947 book, *The Age of Anxiety*. It stands as one of the few books that gave the name to an entire era: the age in which *we* live.

Stress Experiments on Animals

Researchers have been studying the effects of stress on animals for years. The results of so much experimentation cannot be adequately reported in this book. Yet one finding has become so widely accepted, it needs to be expanded upon here: When laboratory animals learn how to prevent pain and stress, they will suffer fewer adverse physical symptoms than animals that cannot prevent the stress.

For instance, laboratory rats can be taught to know when a stressful event is about to occur. Perhaps a ringing bell, or a flashing light, always precedes a mild electric shock. If the animal has the ability to prevent that stressful experience by moving to a safe part of the cage where no shock will be felt, that animal generally experiences few adverse physical symptoms from the overall experience even when it is repeated frequently. On the other hand, if an animal knows a shock is coming but has no way to escape it because there is no safe area, that animal will develop stomach ulcers, brain-tissue damage, and other ills.

Through such research, there is a growing body of evidence to support the theory that our mammalian brains are "hardwired" to deal with stress in ways that can be either nonharmful or harmful, *depending on the actions we are able to take in response to potentially stressful events in our lives.*

Experiments on Humans: Good Stress Boosts the Immune System

If such animal studies offer important lessons about stress's twofold nature, what about experiments involving humans? There is, in fact, a growing body of research to support the hypothesis that our ability to take action in the face of certain stresses actually *improves our health* and ability to resist disease. Conversely there is more evidence suggesting that when we are unable to prevent stress but must passively "take it," we become more susceptible to disease.

In other words, good stress makes us healthier while bad stress tears us down.

One important new study in this area was conducted in 2001 by Jos A. Bosch, a postdoctoral fellow at Ohio State University. Dr. Bosch and his colleagues found that when we have control over the outcomes of stressful events, our immune systems are actually strengthened. When we have no ability to control the outcomes, when we must sit passively and endure stress, our immune response is weakened.

Bosch and his colleagues conducted their experiments on a group of thirty-four volunteers, all male undergraduate students who were exposed to two different stressful experiences. The first experience was a timed test that required the subjects to memorize given material and then take a twelve-minute exam about it. In the second activity, the subjects were shown a twelve-minute video showing surgical procedures, which some might consider gruesome.

What was the difference between these two kinds of acute stresses? In the first, participants were actively engaged in an activity that let them control the outcome. In the second, they had to watch passively. They had no control over what occurred.

To examine the effect of these very different stressful scenarios, Dr. Bosch's researchers measured the concentration of defense proteins known as immunoglobulins in the subjects' saliva. These proteins make up much of the protective outer film of organs, including the lungs. In effect, they serve as the body's first line of defense against disease. Dr. Bosch and his colleagues found that the memory test caused an *increase* in the defensive proteins. In contrast, watching the video had the opposite effect, *lowering* the level of the defensive protein in the saliva.

Such research offers tantalizing evidence that engaging in *positive* stressful experiences is actually good for our physical well-being. It seems likely that research in the years to come will further document this exciting possibility.

"Challenge" vs. "Hindrance" Stress: Findings from Cornell University

Let us return for a moment to the studies mentioned at the start of this chapter, reported in *The Wall Street Journal*. The research in question was conducted in 1998 by Wendy R. Boswell, John W. Boudreau, Marcie A. Cavanaugh, and Mark V. Roehling, researchers at Cornell University's Center for Advanced Human Resource Studies.[*]

---

[*] One of the researchers, Dr. Wendy Boswell, also serves as an assistant management professor at the Mays College & Graduate School of Business at Texas A&M University. The entire research report is available from Cornell as a working paper entitled " 'Challenge' and 'Hindrance,' Related Stress Among U.S. Managers" (Working Paper WP 98-13 from Cornell University's Center for Advanced Human Resource Studies, available online from www.ilr.cornell.edu/cahrs).

The researchers, working in the field of business and human resources, studied a group of 1,886 American managers who were predominantly male (91 percent), white (96 percent) and married (91 percent), with an average age of forty-seven. The respondents worked an average of fifty-six hours a week and earned an average of $164,618 annually.

The purpose of the study was to test this hypothesis:

> **Stresses associated with two kinds of job demands or work circumstances, "challenges" and "hindrances," are distinct phenomena that are differently related to work outcomes . . . results indicate that challenge-related stress is positively related to job satisfaction and negatively related to job search. In contrast, hindrance-related stress is negatively related to job satisfaction and positively related to job search and turnover.**

The researchers determined that there were two kinds of stress:

> **Hindrances are work-related demands or circumstances that tend to constrain or interfere with an individual's work achievement, and which do not tend to be associated with potential gains for the individual. . . . Hindrances result in negative stress or distress (e.g., excessive worry, anguish, frustration, strain).**
>
> **Challenges are work-related demands or circumstances that, although potentially stressful, have associated potential gains for individuals. Potential gains include intrinsic rewards (e.g., satisfaction) and gains that promote work achievement (e.g., achievement related learning, skill development, or demonstration of competence). Work achievement refers to both current job and career success.**

What kind of workplace events were classified as challenges and which as hindrances? Let's take a closer look.

❭ The number of projects on a manager's plate was seen by respondents as a "challenge"; the amount of red tape they had to go through to complete those projects, a "hindrance."

❭ Time pressures were seen as a "challenge"; lack of job security, a "hindrance."

❭ The scope of responsibility was reported as a "challenge"; office politics, a "hindrance."

"On balance, the results provide evidence that challenge-and hindrance-related stresses are distinct phenomena," the researchers reported in the Cornell papers. In her own reporting on the research for Texas A&M University, Dr. Boswell reported her view that challenge stress "propels" employees to work better, while hindrance stress leads to "stalled careers" and eventually to stress-related health problems, including heart disease.

Good and Bad Reactions to Stress

All the research reported above conclusively divides stress into two categories: good stress and bad stress. However, there is another consideration that needs to be mentioned as well: Our individual *reactions* to life's stressful events can be either good or bad.

The fact is, some of us are more susceptible to feelings of anxiety and stress than others. Still more important, as individuals we are sometimes more susceptible to stresses than at other times.

Events that cause us no emotional upset one day can prove deeply troubling the next, seemingly without explanation.

❭ Your boss drops by your office one afternoon and asks, "How's that report coming along?" You experience extreme anxiety after the question and you want to bark back even though you realize you are over-reacting. On another day, the question would have appeared nonthreatening and routine. But for some reason that day, it "puts you over the top."

▶ After dinner one evening, your daughter suddenly remembers that she needs some additional supplies from a craft store so she can build a model of a plant that's due in science class the next day. It's a simple errand, but you inexplicably feel her request is "the straw that breaks" and become very stressed and angry. Your aggravation then blurs into feelings of guilt over your extreme reaction to your kid's simple request, which leads in turn to more stress.

▶ While you're driving to work one morning, another driver cuts you off. You feel flushed, your pulse races, and you get so angry and unsettled that when you arrive at work, people ask you what is wrong. You realize that you are overreacting to a routine event, but that doesn't help. You feel overstressed and unable to calm down.

You can surely add to this short list of routine events that cause extreme stress reactions, seemingly without explanation. Events that "roll off your back" one day seem stressful the next.

Here are some reasons researchers have discovered for why this can happen.

▶ Disrupted sleep patterns, such as getting more or less sleep than usual. Jet lag can contribute too.

▶ An accumulation of stressful events. You handle the first fifty stressful episodes of the day without feeling stressed. But event number fifty-one jolts you into a state of high stress. And it can be an occurrence of very little consequence, like a routine interruption or a phone call from a friend who wants to chat.

▶ Tension that you carry over from other parts of the day. Perhaps you had a stressful day at work and handled it capably but suddenly feel overstressed when arriving at home to spend the evening with your family.

▶ A variety of physical factors, such as changes in diet. High or low blood sugar levels, for example, can cause mood swings that lead to unexplained or excessive emotions.

Understanding these underlying causes of feeling stressed is only the first step. As you follow through on the ideas presented in the rest of this book, you will discover a variety of ways to help you deal with life's many annoyances without losing a sense of control and equilibrium.

We can better understand our reactions to stressful events, and our overreactions too, when we understand that our minds and bodies, over the course of human evolution, have developed complex internal systems to cope with danger.

The Fight or Flight Reaction

Much research has shown that when people become highly stressed, they experience something called the fight or flight reaction. It is the same state that animals enter into when they encounter a physical threat.

It is often said that when we experience the fight or flight reaction, we become just like our cavemen or cavewomen forebears who were confronting saber-toothed tigers or other threats in the wild. We had to fight or escape from danger, even "kill or be killed." Today those reactions remain "hardwired" into our brains.

Once the reaction triggers, the body readies itself to meet the physical demands of conflict or escape. Our heart rate rises, adrenaline is released, blood pressure rises, our muscles become tense, our arteries dilate, our perspiration increases, and our livers release glucose that will fuel our exertions. Our bodies and metabolisms become primed.

Of course, flight or fight is an appropriate response when we are facing genuine physical danger. Many researchers, however, have determined that people today, especially those who are habitually stressed, enter into the state too frequently, even when a perceived threat is not life-menacing at all.

If you're among those who overreact to stress in this way, your brain, in response to even small threats, jumps to send danger signals to your body. You find yourself going into high alert when the phone rings, a car horn honks, or your spouse says, "Honey, there's something I need to ask you about."

Frequent excursions into flight or fight territory are extremely unhealthy. Prolonged exposure to adrenaline alone can adversely affect the normal functioning of the liver, kidneys, and other organs. People who have entered into this dangerous psychological/physical territory need help often through counseling, medication, or other stress-reduction techniques such as meditation or biofeedback, which are sometimes helpful.

Yet help is at hand. As we'll discover in the chapters ahead, we can stop living at the mercy of the extreme reactions to stress that we've learned, even those that have been built into our brains over the course of human evolution.

In the pages that follow, we'll consider our individual stresses in a new way and begin to divide the good from the bad.

At this point, please turn to pages 157–172 at the end of this book and complete your Personal Stress Inventory worksheet. By answering its two hundred questions, you will have a clearer idea of where your personal stresses lie. It's information you will need as you process your stress.

2

LEARNING TO LOOK
AT STRESS IN A NEW WAY

As you discovered while completing your Personal Stress Inventory, stresses come in all shapes and sizes, from simple to complex, from small to large.

In this chapter you will begin to understand and process the results of your Personal Stress Inventory. As you think about each of the stresses you discovered, how will you decide which are bad, which good?

It will take a little time, since many stresses won't reveal their true nature as good or bad until you begin to work on them. Let's start that process by looking critically at seven essential differences between good stresses and bad.

Remember, the following laws are general guidelines I have developed after conducting extensive research into the topic of stress. They are not infallible. As you use these rules to decide which of your personal stresses are good or bad, you might discover that some of your stresses are too complex to fit easily within them. If you're about to break off a troubled love relationship and you can predict your partner will be hurt and not forgive you, for example, you may be dealing with a stress that doesn't comfortably conform to Rule 6—"Good stresses improve our relationships with other people. Bad stresses make relationships worse." Still, you know that breaking off the relationship will be a good thing and produce positive results even though someone else might be upset by the actions you are about to take.

But more often than not, these rules will provide needed

insight into which stresses are bad in your life and which will produce positive outcomes when you take action on them. Let's take a closer look.

The Seven Good Stress or Bad Stress Laws

1: We exert a high level of control over the outcomes of good stresses. With bad stresses, we enjoy little influence over what will happen.

Perhaps you're feeling stressed about a job review next week. No doubt about it, it promises to be a highly stressful event. But at the same time, you can take action to control the outcome. You could document the costs you've cut since your last review, for example, and be ready to highlight that information during your review. Or you might ask your customers to provide testimonials about the excellent service you've been providing. In other words, you can control the outcome by taking action.

With bad stress, you are at a loss to exert control. Let's say you're working for a company that is about to be acquired. What will your new job be? Will you even *have* a job? What will happen to your current projects, your staff, your computer, your office? Until you gain some knowledge about what is about to take place, you have little way to control something critical in your life. Things might get better, they might get worse, but for the moment you are living with bad stress.

2: We experience positive feelings when we process good stress. When bad stresses leave our lives, negative or ambivalent feelings follow.

Perhaps you're stressed about applying for a loan to pay for your kid's first year of college. You worry that the process will be unpleasant, that your application might get turned down, that the monthly payments you'll have to make will be unbearable. But after you go to the loan officer, you feel relieved. You have now armed yourself with the knowledge that you need to dispel your fears and make some sound decisions about college finances. As a result, you experience a new sense of relief and control. Or perhaps you felt anguished about whether or not to apply for a certain job, then elated when you tried and were hired. Good stresses went away, leaving good feelings behind.

Bad stress, in contrast, dissipates in less positive ways. Your siblings have been struggling over the decision to place an ailing parent in an extended-care facility. After you make the best decision possible, select a nursing home, and decide to move ahead, you might experience some good feelings but also nagging doubts and guilt about whether you did the right thing.

Or maybe you're about to make the difficult decision to sell the home where you grew up, or where you raised your family. Even though you realize that selling the place is the most rational course, the actions you are about to take will not be happy ones. You know negative feelings and doubts will result, possibly long-lasting ones.

If you are considering one stress in your life and trying to apply this yardstick, you may be asking the question "This law of stress is interesting, but how can I know how a particular stress will dissipate until I act upon it?" Of course, you are right to ask this question. There is no way to accurately predict how a stress will disappear until you take steps to chase it away. You can, however, take a moment to ask the question, "How would I feel if I took steps to resolve this problem?"

Applying that simple yardstick can provide new insights into which of the life stresses you discovered in the Personal Stress Inventory are good and which bad.

3: Good stresses help us achieve positive goals. Bad stresses offer no desirable outcomes.

Having discussions with your husband or wife about all the expensive renovations you're planning for your home might seem to be a stressful event. So might making a sales call to an important potential client. Both these events appear filled with anxiety. Yet when you take a closer look, you find they embody specific goals and desirable outcomes. Perhaps with some careful planning, you and your spouse really can budget enough money to fix up your home the way you would like. If you are a salesperson, you might not make the sale. Then again, you *might*. There will be an end to the anxiety, which will dissipate as issues are resolved.

In sharp contrast, bad stresses don't offer opportunities to make personal progress. Let's say, for example, that you are dealing with a teenage child who is rebellious, uncontrollable, angry at you, and uncommunicative about what he or she is doing when you are not there to watch. Of course, there is an outcome you can envision, deep in the distance. Time will move on and somehow the problem will improve and be dissipated. Yet even the best strategies you can devise for the problem (to be a good parent, to be confrontational, to try to understand, etc.) have little apparent power to resolve the problem directly. You are swimming in a pool of irremovable anxiety.

4: We feel eager when anticipating the work we need to do to process our good stresses. When facing bad stresses, we experience feelings of exhaustion and avoidance.

This distinction can be seen in many areas of life where we are dealing with good stress. You might be planning an important client presentation at work. Or you might be running for president of your high school class. At the moment you are sitting just offstage, about to make the speech that will determine the outcome. Are you stressed in these situations? Scared too? Of course you are. But at the same time, you feel a sense of positive energy, excitement, and challenge. Through your stress you are living more fully.

Bad stresses are far different. Perhaps you're driving to your son's soccer game, knowing that you are about to have a confrontation with his belligerent coach about whether your boy will be allowed to take the field. It's possible that the confrontation will turn out to be a good stress if things might turn out better than you expect and good outcomes might result. But chances are that you will emerge from the showdown with new problems to solve and new stresses to process. You might even feel the attraction of the flight side of the fight or flight syndrome. You want only to avoid the situation and get away.

It's interesting to note that many unhappy lives are deeply rooted in avoiding bad stresses. The pattern may start when an individual indulges the natural desire to avoid one or two difficult problems and from there, it infects all of life's important, positive challenges. Healthy patterns of dealing with good stresses and challenges exert the opposite effect. People who have dealt with stresses and obstacles in healthy ways tend to be more active, confident, energetic. In short, they are better able to resiliently deal with the new challenges that life places in their path.

5: Good stresses make us grow. Bad stresses box us in.

This principle is especially evident at work. When we're lucky enough to have jobs that offer good stresses, such as opportunities to advance and learn, we expand our abilities and move ahead with our careers. Often, we move upward within our organizations.

If, in contrast, we are offered only bad stresses (repetitive tasks, limited leeway to think for ourselves, pointless frictions with customers or colleagues), we sense that we have nowhere to go. Our bad stress leads to stagnation. It is possible to make the situation better, as we'll discover in the final chapters of this book. But doing so means taking action to either reinvent the situation or, in some cases, escaping the situation entirely and moving to a better place.

6: Good stresses improve our relationships with other people. Bad stresses make relationships worse.

We see this principle at work in many of life's good-but-stressful activities, such as:

▶ making a decision with your family about which new home to buy
▶ picking a private school for one of your children
▶ working with your congregation to recruit a new minister, rabbi, imam or priest as your spiritual leader

Are such activities difficult and stressful? Yes! There will be frictions and disagreements along the way. But they generally offer the opportunity to grow closer to other people as you work with them in the problem-solving process.

On the opposite pole, dealing with bad stresses usually fosters feelings of alienation, estrangement or even irreconcilable rifts between you and others.

You and your divorcing spouse are in conflict over child custody. Even if fair decisions are made, your relationship with your former spouse (and possibly your new spouse or partner as well) will suffer. Most important, your relationship with your children might well become destabilized. This is bad stress at its worst!

Your business partner wants to take your company in one direction, and you do not agree. Because your views are opposed and seemingly irreconcilable, bad feelings are apt to result even if you and your partner decide to part ways.

In summary, groups of people who are engaged in good-but-stressful pursuits experience feelings of camaraderie. Groups of people who are dealing with bad stresses bicker and disagree. It is a good example of the difference between *challenge* and *hindrance* stress.

7: Processing any stress, whether good or bad, requires action on our part.

No good or bad stress will reveal its true nature until you invest work and energy to process it. In other words, laziness won't cut it, or simply waiting around to see what will happen when and if a stressful problem goes away.

Yet there is a particular payoff when we are working hard to process our stresses. We develop a level of personal resilience that makes our lives fuller, more accomplished, and more rewarding.

In the end, processing good stress can even become, as Hans Selye stated, "the spice of life."

Looking at the 7 Rules in a Different Way:

Good Stress or Bad Stress Checklist

Good stress	*Bad stress*
■ Offers visible rewards	■ Has no desirable outcomes in sight
■ Brings people together	■ Drives people apart
■ Lets you develop and grow	■ Limits you
■ Boosts self-esteem	■ Makes you feel worse about yourself
■ Ends with resolution	■ Merges into new conflicts and problems
■ Changes into something good when relieved	■ Becomes something bad when relieved
■ Opens up new possibilities when resolved	■ Is dead-ended
■ Results in high achievement	■ Lowers personal standards
■ Breeds optimism	■ Causes negativism and defeatist attitudes

Make a preliminary decision about which of your stresses are good or bad.

TURN to the scoring section at the end of your Personal Stress Inventory, where you listed your "highly stressful" personal stresses. Based on the good stress or bad stress laws in this chapter and the chart above, tentatively divide them into two lists under each category:

- Stresses which you expect to be good stresses, based on those rules
- Stresses which you suspect might be bad

Some stresses will clearly fall into good or bad. Others require further work and processing from you before they reveal their true nature. The point is, you are now beginning to process your major life stresses. Use the grid below to track your progress in deciding which of your stresses are good and which bad. Answer each question by filling in the number from the Personal Stress Inventory that applies.

Global/National Issues

Which of my "highly stressful" responses in this category might turn out to be good stresses?_____

Which of my "highly stressful" responses might turn out to be bad?_____

Home Life and Routines

Which of my "highly stressful" responses in this category might turn out to be good stresses?_____

Which of my "highly stressful" responses might turn out to be bad?_____

Parenting

Which of my "highly stressful" responses in this category
 might turn out to be good stresses?_____

Which of my "highly stressful" responses might turn out to
 be bad?_____

Marriage/Love Relationships

Which of my "highly stressful" responses in this category
 might turn out to be good stresses?_____

Which of my "highly stressful" responses might turn out to
 be bad?_____

Other Family Relationships

Which of my "highly stressful" responses in this category
 might turn out to be good stresses?_____

Which of my "highly stressful" responses might turn out to
 be bad?_____

Finances

Which of my "highly stressful" responses in this category
 might turn out to be good stresses?_____

Which of my "highly stressful" responses might turn out to
 be bad?_____

Job and Career

Which of my "highly stressful" responses in this category
 might turn out to be good stresses?_____

Which of my "highly stressful" responses might turn out to
 be bad?_____

Health

Which of my "highly stressful" responses in this category
 might turn out to be good stresses?_____

Which of my "highly stressful" responses might turn out to
 be bad?_____

Overriding Personal Issues

Which of my "highly stressful" responses in this category
   might turn out to be good stresses?_____

Which of my "highly stressful" responses might turn out to
   be bad?_____

PART II

Making the Most of Good Stress

The realization that good stress exists offers us the opportunity to move confidently forward in many areas of our lives that we previously perceived as merely stressful, and therefore stalled.

In this section we will explore good stress in many of its guises. We will encounter good stresses that reveal their beneficial nature at once, as soon as we stop to ask "Is this stress actually beneficial to me?"

We will also explore another category of good stresses: Stresses that we *believed* were bad but which turn out to be good when we take action on them.

3

UNCOVERING THE
GOOD STRESSES IN YOUR LIFE

While reading Chapters 1 and 2 you probably discovered you were habitually misclassifying many potentially good stresses in your life as bad.

As a result, you may have cut off many of the opportunities good stress can offer you, including chances to grow, solve problems, cooperate better with people, and more.

At this point I'd like to pause to consider a fundamental question about stress. Why do we tend to see all our stresses as bad and miss their potential benefits? Why don't we already know that many stressful pursuits offer us a high payback in life? I don't know all the answers to those questions, of course, but here are some that seem logical.

We've been conditioned to think all stress is bad. Today we are learning that branding all stress as bad doesn't make any sense. However, for the last half century newspaper articles, television shows, and books have taught us that all tension is bad for us. We've learned our lessons well. We accept the notion that stress and tension will cause physical problems and shorten our lives.

It takes a conscious effort to remind ourselves that the tensions we are experiencing might be either good or bad. If you and your spouse are experiencing frictions about money, for example, you've probably assumed that you have hit an area that can pose very grave danger to your relationship. Talking about money could trigger an argument, years of conflict, even divorce! Such thinking, of course, is flawed. If your relationship is sound, talking about sensitive issues in the right way will actually *strengthen* your relationship. You are dealing with good stress here, directing you toward an area that needs attention if your relationship is to grow stronger. (As we will see in Chapter 10, stresses in our relationships often help us discover areas where we can grow closer to loved ones.) We need to change the way we think about stress.

We suffer from the straw-that-breaks syndrome. As we have already observed, the pace of our lives can cause us to snap into the fight or flight state with too little provocation. We handle dozens of stressful events all day long, but then one comes along and pushes us "over the edge" into uncontrollable stress. At work, it might be something completely routine, such as a call from a colleague who asks "Can we meet at ten tomorrow morning instead of noon?" Or when you arrive home for supper, your boyfriend or girlfriend mentions that your cat seems to be getting sick and one of you needs to take the next morning off to pay a call to the veterinarian. These are not life-threatening events such as car accidents, heart attacks, or fires that break out in the home. Yet if they happen to serve as the straws that break, they catapult us into extreme stress anyway.

If we become chronic sufferers of this syndrome, we can even train our biological clocks to enter into high alert at specific times of the day. Perhaps we experience one event late every morning at work that gets our brains firing in high-stress mode for the rest of the day. Or when we arrive home each evening, we overreact to something a family member says and we stay upset for hours. If no real crisis triggers the response, we create one to fill our need for one. All the new stresses we encounter and create flow into one large, undifferentiated mash of anxiety from which we cannot escape. We lose the ability to see anything good in the routine events that life brings our way.

We catastrophize. Instead of seeing stresses for what they are, we overreact and peg them as signs of bigger problems.

When your child brings home a French quiz with an uncharacteristically low grade of C-, you overreact and see that as the first sign of major troubles ahead in school. Or when a customer calls to say a piece of equipment she leased from you needs service, you feel certain that you are about to lose the entire account.

When we fall victim to catastrophizing's lure, insignificant events take on major importance, while the things that matter the most to us get put aside and ignored. We become so mired in thinking that everything is wrong that we lose perspective on everything that is going well in our lives.

Yet there are some effective, immediate remedies to our learned tendency to overreact to stress. Instead of directing blame at ourselves because stress is "wrong" or because we are not able to "handle it well," we can utilize the following tools to make the situation better.

Serve as Your Own Emotional Gatekeeper

When you find yourself overreacting to a new stress (your pulse quickens, your breathing speeds, you feel flushed), remind yourself to take a moment to ask whether you are dealing appropriately with the event that triggered the symptoms you are feeling. Are you reacting irrationally?

The key is to learn to act as your own emotional gatekeeper, a keen self-observer who continually evaluates incoming stresses to determine which are genuinely serious and which are not. As an aid in this process, it can be helpful to imagine a "stress gauge" with a needle that swings upward through zones marked "small stress," "moderate stress," and "major stress." Whenever you encounter a new stress, imagine the face of your stress gauge and ask "Okay, how high should this problem cause the needle to go?"

Armed with this objective tool (or with any other stress-monitoring tool you personally create), you will find that most of the new stresses that come your way will fall into the "small" or "moderate" stress categories, which is precisely where they belong. You will often see that you have been overreacting to many stresses that are not so threatening at all.

❱ When the chairperson of your parent-teacher organization calls and asks you to prepare dessert instead of a casserole for a meeting the next day, that is not a life-threatening calamity. It's an annoyance, but you can handle it.

❱ When you walk into a class and learn that you'll be taking a surprise quiz, you're a bit put off and concerned. But this stress, annoying though it might be, still doesn't represent anything life-threatening. It might even offer an opportunity to do very well.

❱ When your car repair shop calls to tell you the "little rattle" you heard was actually a loose main crankshaft bearing that's going to cost $1,100 to repair, the imaginary needle on your stress gauge might sweep high up into the "major stress" zone. Yet will it stay there? Probably not. Your stress, though serious, is not a life-threatening event.

❱ When your husband brings home a bundle of mint leaves instead of basil for you to use in preparing pesto for the evening pasta entree, you might be tempted to bark at him that the meal is "ruined." But when you act as your own personal stress gatekeeper, you will know at once that it is a minor problem that merits only a minor degree of annoyance on your part. You can probably even *laugh* about it.

By evaluating and weighing our incoming stresses, we begin to develop the perspective that we need to differentiate good stresses from bad.

Practice "Opportunity Thinking"

Dr. Richard Shoup, a psychotherapist who wrote the book *Take Control of Your Life* with me several years ago, states that "opportunity thinking" can serve as an effective antidote to overreacting to life's routine events.

"Opportunities often arise from random occurrences," Dr. Shoup explains, "and that's a fascinating reality if we stop to think about it. With the right outlook, we can turn chaotic events into opportunities."

Here are some of Dr. Shoup's suggestions for putting opportunity thinking into practice:

Remind yourself that seemingly mundane events often contain hidden opportunities. Every day is filled with events and incoming information. Yet certain things that come our way are different from the rest. They represent *opportunities*. If we learn to look out for them, we can seize them and turn them to our advantage. When an important client calls and wants to initiate a serious discussion, for example, we can see that as a threat. But it might also represent an opportunity to resolve problems, improve service, or reach other worthwhile goals. Whether it is a bad stress or a good stress might actually depend on our expectations.

Look for opportunities in events that appear threatening at first glance. If you walk into a routine meeting and the company president is unexpectedly sitting there, for example, your first reaction might be to jump into full fight or flight mode. But the presence of this man or woman at the meeting might actually present a valuable opportunity to show your abilities, to bring up a concern that is weighing on your colleagues, or excel in some other way.

Learn to be playful and *enjoy* some parts of chaos. Of course, that can be a tall order in today's hectic world. Yet with a playful outlook, the chaos itself (the ringing phones, interruptions, sudden emergencies) can be fascinating and even fun. We become almost like goalies in a hockey game. A lot of things are flying our way at once, yet we discover we can deal with them all as we stay tuned to the larger strategies that are part of the game.

In short, we need to stay tuned for the opportunities that good stress can bring. Often, circumstances that seem to be pushing us beyond our limits actually represent good stresses, not bad. When we realize that it is possible to become masters of incoming stresses instead of victims, we learn to live in a higher way.

Exercise

Spend a day time-warping all stressful events.

FOR one day, simply delay all the stressful events that intrude on you.

When the paper hanger unexpectedly calls to say he can start putting new wallpaper in your living room tomorrow and you start to "freak out" about getting everything ready, ask him to start two days later.

When Paul, your least favorite colleague, calls and says, "Can I see you right away?" and you feel your blood pressure rise, say, "No, not now, but at ten tomorrow morning."

These time changes may appear inconsequential. Yet when we "time-warp" stressful events, interesting things begin to happen. We realize we have more control over our schedules than we often utilize. We do not live at the beck and call of other people. By the end of the day, we have also gained a better perspective about the events that were unsettling us. ("I allowed myself to get so stressed out about a meeting with Paul? Why?")

The result can be the realization that we have more control that we might expect over what stresses us and what does not. As noted at the outset of this book, part of what makes stresses good or bad is not contained in the stresses themselves but in our *reaction* to them. When we consciously learn to control that, we have gained an edge.

4

USING GOOD STRESS
TO PERFORM AT YOUR BEST

Life sometimes requires us to perform at our best before the eyes of other people. We have speeches and presentations to give, athletic contests we'd like to win, plays to appear in, solos to sing in church or at school, not to mention important life rituals like our weddings, our children's weddings, confirmations, bar and bat mitzvahs. And on the list goes.

In this chapter we'll explore ways to use the natural nervousness that accompanies such events to perform better. In other words, we will explore ways to unlock the good stress that lies hidden within performance-related events that frighten us. If, however, you have an acute problem with performance anxiety (if you feel completely panicked and "frozen" before certain tasks you often perform in your life or work), it might be a good idea to seek the help of a qualified therapist who can offer help tailored to particular needs. The advice in this book cannot be customized sufficiently to meet your individual issues.

Unlocking the Good Stress
in Performance Anxiety

You have certainly encountered situations when tension and stress enabled you to reach a higher level of performance or enjoyment than you could have achieved otherwise. Perhaps you felt nervous before giving an important talk. Yet as you began, your agitation transformed into positive energy. You exceeded your own expectations and did a wonderful job.

Or perhaps you were organizing an important fund-raising event at your place of worship, your kids' school, or elsewhere. The tension that built up in the weeks ahead spurred you to coordinate the work of a large group of people. Through the unpleasant prodding of stress, you uncovered leadership abilities in yourself that you hadn't discovered before. And the results were excellent.

The release of good stress often allows us to reach new levels of satisfaction, even in tasks we were dreading. Yet there is a darker side to performance-related stress too.

You have probably encountered situations when your nervousness before an important event caused you to perform at a *lower* level than you might have done without all that nervousness.

When you stood up to the microphone to make your talk, you sweated uncontrollably and your voice cracked. Through your whole talk you were concerned only with controlling your nervousness. As a result, you really *didn't* do your best. Or perhaps your nervousness on the day of your college baseball playoffs caused you to make some uncharacteristic mistakes in the field.

In such situations, our ability to unlock the good opportunities inherent in high-stakes situations can be lost. Our anxiety lapses over into bad stress and, on the spot, we can find no simple remedy.

How can we manage life's performance-tied stressful situations capably so we enjoy good stress instead of stalling in the bad? The answer lies in finding ways to understand, and combat, the specific fears and anxieties that are most likely to strike us.

The Fear that Something Will Go Wrong

"Catastrophizing" is a natural mental process we all engage in before high-stakes events. Fears take over and increase the odds that we really will be immobilized if something unexpected occurs.

❯ When you take your driver's road test, you will completely bungle parallel parking and fail to get your license.

❯ The florist will fail to deliver the flowers for your daughter's confirmation luncheon and the tables will look bare and awful.

❯ Midway through the keynote speech you are giving at a major convention, a breeze will suddenly blow away your note cards and you will have to scramble around the room to collect them.

❯ People will not even giggle at the jokes you've written into the toast you will make at your best friend's wedding.

You can surely add your own items to the above list, based on personal experiences. Yet there is a fallacy at the root of such worries, the belief that if one thing goes wrong, *everything else* will then go wrong too.

It's a "house of cards" scenario that makes whatever you are about to do appear much more risky than it really is.

One effective way to counter this problem is to stage rehearsals in which you make sure things really *do* go wrong, just to prove to yourself that miscues and mistakes don't have the power to ruin your performance.

Some exercises to try:

❯ If you're worried about an upcoming presentation, ask a friend to sit in on a rehearsal. Invite her to do anything possible to disrupt your talk. She can pepper you with hostile questions, run up and toss your notes on the floor, unplug your sound system. Or if you are worried about what might happen if you suddenly lost your notes before your talk, go to the podium empty-handed and see what happens when you have to "wing it." You will see that the events you are imagining really don't have the power to stop you cold.

▶ If you're obsessing that you will bungle the parallel-parking phase of your driving test, go to a vacant parking lot on a quiet afternoon and perform all the steps of the driving test you can think of, then intentionally fail to parallel park well. Put up some traffic cones, knock them down, and enjoy the sound. This exercise will show you all the things you in reality do well, and also remind you that parallel parking is only a small part of the overall test you are about to take.

▶ If you are about to play a piano piece in a class recital and worry about having a memory lapse, have a special rehearsal where one of your friends yells "stop!" three or four times as you play your piece (or set the alarm on a digital watch to ring every thirty seconds and stop every time it goes off). After a few such experiments, you will see that being forced to stop and then resume at unexpected times can't completely derail your performance. The worst memory lapse will cause one percent of your overall performance to be somewhat substandard. That's not a complete catastrophe by any means.

When you actually rehearsed your imagined catastrophes, they will no longer hold great fear for you. They are now a part of your routine. If things go wrong, you now know how to deal with them flexibly and keep moving ahead.

The Fear that Nerves Will Keep You from Doing Your Best

At the heart of this concern lies the simple fact that you are comparing your "best" performance (possibly the one you achieved in practicing your speech in your hotel room, or with your team in the final practice before a big game) to the imaginary one that will occur at the stress-inducing event itself. You start to worry about it.

How can you ever repeat your best performance, which you achieved in practice, at the event itself?

This fear, though based on an exaggeration ("If I don't perform perfectly, my performance won't be any good") does have a basis in reality. No matter how much you practice your sales pitch, your piano sonata, or your fast ball, your performance at the event itself really will not be precisely the same. Nerves or other factors really *will* cause your actual performance to be different. You might do better, you might do worse. Only time will tell.

Yet you can actually rehearse *nerves* and learn that bad as they are, they lack the power to completely destroy what you will achieve.

Dr. Don Greene, a psychotherapist and author of an excellent book *Fight Your Fear and Win,* is a specialist who helps performing artists and athletes overcome extreme nervousness. He has taught his techniques to the U. S. Olympic Diving Team, to classical pianists, and to opera singers who "freeze" before auditions. The following exercise developed by Dr. Greene is extremely helpful in reducing pre-performance nerves.

Dr. Greene asks people who suffer from acute nerves to actually run up a few flights of stairs to simulate a nervous state. For example, a pianist will run up those stairs, race to a piano, sit down, and start to play. In this exercise, people who suffer from performance anxiety discover they really can learn to perform capably, even with sweaty palms, a pounding heart, and heavy breathing. As they pant and shake, they can "center" by taking some deep breaths and soldier on until they regain control of themselves. Because they know the sensation of starting a performance with extreme stress (and moving ahead anyway), they have mastered a behavior pattern that transfers directly to succeeding in their stressful activity.

Again, by rehearsing the worst, they have increased the odds of performing at their best.

"Fear Within a Fear," Obsessing that You Can't Calm Down

You have certainly encountered this problem. Just before you stepped up before the committee to defend your doctoral dissertation, or laced up your ice skates before an important figure-skating competition, your nervousness made you say, "I have to relax, I need to calm down."

If you succumb to this fear, you are setting up false expectations. It is virtually impossible to "calm down" before high-stakes activities unless you are a master athlete, musician, or other professional who engages in high-stakes activities so often that they have become completely routine for you. Even then, you will rarely enter into such activities in a completely relaxed way; you will instead use nervousness to be energized and in control.

Relaxation is actually a false goal. In fact, we are indulging in self-sabotage by telling ourselves "I can do well only if I feel calm." The real goal should be to channel your excess energy so that it can boost your performance, not sabotage it.

It takes practice, but it can be done.

Direct your nervous energy toward a small, highly focused goal. The tennis pro who runs into mid-match trouble when facing a hard-charging opponent might consciously forget there's an opponent on the other side of the net and concentrate all his nervous energy on the simple act of returning the ball. (He can therefore concentrate on controlling the elements of his *own* game, not the one dictated by the opponent. That's a stronger psychological position.) Or a French horn player who must perform a difficult solo passage in a symphony knows she will not do her best if she allows herself to concentrate on *everything*: the audience sitting in the hall, the frown on the conductor's face, the player in the next chair who thinks *he* should be playing the solo instead of her. So she shuts out all those secondary concerns and directs all her energy at something well defined and simple that she can control, such as the way her lips meet inside the mouthpiece as she starts the first note or the shape of the first musical phrase in her solo.

Practice the art of "steadying up" by learning to recover when nerves intrude. Like other exercises recommended in this chapter, you can intentionally allow things to go wrong in practice and discover the specific skills needed to make them come right again. If you are worried that you will be too nervous to serve the volleyball well in an upcoming tournament, tell your teammates at one practice that you will intentionally serve badly four or five times, then practice the skills needed to pull your serve back onto the court and serve well afterward. Or if you are obsessing about the possibility that your knees will be knocking when you get up to deliver a toast at your brother's wedding, do some deep knee bends and then rehearse giving your toast so you can master the sensation of delivering it on unsteady legs.

Through such exercises, you will see that nerves can alter your performance but that you can direct the energy they bring to do even better than you might have expected.

Remember, Butterflies Are Good

There is still another tie between nerves and peak performance. The "butterflies" that may occur when you are attempting something really significant can be a certain indicator that you are encountering good stress. Terrie Williams, a vibrant woman who is a major force in the world of public relations, says she has actually learned to *welcome* butterflies as an important indication that she is attempting something that promises to stretch her into new realms of responsibility.

She says that when she is waiting for an important meeting to begin, jitters in her stomach offer a reliable indication that she is doing just what she should be doing: moving her life to a higher level.

Williams, whose firm represents such clients as Time Warner, the National Basketball Association, Johnnie Cochran, and Lionel Ritchie, knows what she is talking about.

A life without butterflies, she says, means not risking enough. That's advice that serves as a testament to the transforming power of good stress in our lives.

Exercise

Master the recurring high-stress events in your life.

THE first step in this exercise is to identify the repetitive activities in your life that cause you to experience a level of performance anxiety: the high-stakes public activities that stand out from the rest of what you do. A review of the results of your Personal Stress Inventory should give you an immediate list of acute performance-related stressors such as these:

- "Psyching up" for the monthly visit that the CEO and company president make to the assembly line where you work
- Coaching games for your son's basketball league
- Giving annual performance reviews to the members of your staff
- Making sales pitches to potential new clients

Create a personal list of these "high stressors" and direct special attention to unlocking the good stress they contain by processing them with the approaches recommended in this chapter.

Practice that sales presentation aloud and invite a member of your staff to interrupt and sabotage you, for example. Or as you step into the gym as a coach before one of your son's games, mentally shut out the yells from the sidelines and direct all your nervous tension at the basics of what each of your players should be doing.

When you reduce the negative sensations of stress that you habitually tie to such high-stakes activities, you will learn to unlock the good stress that's hidden in them.

5

TAPPING GOOD STRESS
TO GET INTO FLOW

Flow can occur only in stressful situations. Suddenly the pressure melts away as we realize that a difficult task is far easier than we expected. We realize we've been locking horns with good stress without recognizing it.

All of us have entered into a state of flow. This wonderful sensation, that we are excelling at a complex task with remarkable ease, can occur when we least expect it. We suddenly see that activities we were dreading were not negative at all. In fact, they were chances to enjoy life at a higher level and perform in new and more effective ways.

Flow can happen when we are driving, playing a game of tennis, or tackling a complex task at work.

Just what is flow? It is a state first defined by a psychologist, Dr. Mihaly Csikszentmihaltyi. In his book *Flow: The Psychology of Optimal Experience*, Dr. Csikszentmihaltyi describes it this way:

> . . . a sense that one's skills are adequate to cope with the challenges at hand, in a goal-directed, rule-bound action system that provides clear clues as to how well one is performing. Concentration is so intense that there is no attention left over to think about anything irrelevant, or to worry about problems. Self-consciousness disappears, and the sense of times becomes distorted. An activity that produces such experiences is so gratifying that people are willing to do it for its own sake, with lit-

tle concern for what they will get out of it, even when it is difficult, or dangerous.

The Link Between Stress and Flow

Remarkably, the sensation of flow can occur *only* in stressful situations. We feel immediate relief when a task we have been avoiding turns out to be easier than we expected. At such times, we can even become impressed with our own abilities.

That is a pleasant surprise. However, most of us are soon frustrated when we see that flow will not start whenever we want it to. When we confront stressful tasks, we try to get flow to "kick in" and help us through, and it simply will not.

Why won't flow come to help us whenever we want? Because some very specific elements need to be in place before true flow can start.

An appropriate level of mastery must be present. Mastery can be defined as an individual's ability to perform capably within the context of a task's rules and constraints. Machinists who have mastered their ability to operate high-precision equipment often get into flow, as do professional drivers and golf players. Yet for flow to occur, your level of mastery must be matched to the task. If you have never touch-typed before, for example, and are striving to write a work of fiction for the first time, you will probably be excluded from a state of flow. If you are a tennis player of intermediate ability, you will sometimes be able to enter into a state of flow when playing against another player whose skills approximate your own. If you play against Pete Sampras or one of the Williams sisters, all bets are off.

There have to be rules, sometimes, a great many. Consider classical musicians who must play the written notes as they perform, or ballet dancers who must follow the rhythms of the music as well as the choreographer's steps. Yet we also know that these people are among the most likely to enter into a state of flow as they perform. Rules *help* them.

There must be stress and pressure. People who use the flow state to perform at a high level report that they *need* deadlines, *need* demands, *need* intense competition to do their best. There are few clearer depictions of the rewards of good stress.

Getting into Flow When You Need To

In light of the above considerations, how can you use flow to increase your sense of easy control over life's difficult tasks? Here are some steps to follow.

Make sure your skills are up to the task at hand. As noted, flow will elude you when you attempt tasks that exceed your skills and abilities. For this reason, it can be worthwhile to add to your repertoire of needed skills in the areas where you would most like to benefit from flow. If you need to use a computer for many tasks at work and would like to increase the likelihood that you will get into flow in those tasks, take the computer training you need to bring those skills up to par. Or if woodworking is your hobby and you would like to experience much more joy from the pursuit, it might be a good idea to take some classes. The more developed your skills become, the more often flow will occur.

Stay active. That sounds like a basic piece of advice. And, of course, it is. Procrastination is one of greatest impediments to flow. Unless we take that first step and jump into the activity we are dreading, we have no way of gaining the sense that we have control over it. In some cases, taking that first step is really all that is needed to unlock positive stress and enter into a state of flow.

Practice. That one word says it all. It's the most effective way to improve skills to the point where flow occurs naturally and easily. The greatest athletes, actors, musicians, fighter pilots, orators, all practice. And if they can do it, we can too.

Break large tasks down into smaller parts and attack them separately. When we narrow our focus to a small part of a large process, we increase the likelihood of flow. For example, it can be highly effective to say "I will invest thirty minutes outlining my term paper this afternoon, but I won't start writing it until tomorrow." Such limitations bring greater focus and results.

Try achieving flow at different training stages. If you are an amateur violinist beginning to play chamber music, find some playing partners whose skills approximate your own. You can then experience a sensation of flow that you can carry upward to your next level of mastery. The joy of flow, whenever it can be achieved, speeds learning and increases your motivation to move ahead much more than entering into situations that are above your head.

Assemble the tools you need to support your effort. They might be low tech (sharp new chisels if you are a wood-carver), medium tech (a small collection of good lenses if you are a photographer), or high tech (the latest script-writing software if you are writing a screenplay). Tools that are well matched to your level of competence trigger flow. Unmatched tools hold you back or frustrate you.

Concentrate. When you direct your mind concertedly toward an activity, you raise the process to a higher level and increase the likelihood that a state of flow will occur. Sometimes, you might nearly have to force yourself to direct your mind in this way. It can be a struggle until you begin to experience the rewards.

Eliminate interruptions. Ringing phones, kids running in to ask for homework help, a group of friends coming over in a half hour for a game of cards—such intrusions usually destroy any chance of entering into a state of flow. For this reason, you may want to set aside an afternoon to tackle a high-stakes task. Turn off the ringer on your phone and let your answering machine get the calls. You should even shut off the radio and work in silence.

Set specific challenges for yourself. Flow will rarely begin if you just set time aside to "see what happens." Instead, set up positive expectations such as "I will take my sketch pad to the mountain and come back with three finished drawings of spring flowers." The goal should be challenging, and it should be motivational. When you come home carrying those sketches, you will know you have accomplished something that moves you closer to a significant goal or achievement. You might have even glimpsed what it means to be in flow.

Become a keen observer of events or obstacles that take you out of the flow state. Some people report that a cluttered desk distracts them and prevents flow, for example. Others report that they must return all outstanding phone calls before they start on an important project. Otherwise they feel too distracted to concentrate. Observe yourself and remove whatever stops you.

Exercise

Break a large project down and experience flow.

SELECT one large, complex project, preferably one you have been delaying or dreading. Then attack it in this unusual way.

Take a stack of index cards. Without thinking too hard, write any step from your project on one index card. Then take another index card and write another step on that card. Continue until you cannot think of any more steps. You will soon have completed your complete project "deck."

Spread all the cards out on a table where you can see what is written on them. Pick up the card that represents the step you'd enjoy doing first. Then pick up the card that represents the second most enjoyable, and so on. Continue picking up all the cards until they are in a logical order. The deck has now become your project outline.

Attacking your intimidating project in this way, by first completing the part of it that motivates you most strongly, will initiate a sense of flow that can then be carried over to the other phases.

Whether your goal is to write a novel or prepare your own taxes, you'll feel the negative sensations of bad stress melt away and the positive emotions that accompany the release of good stress begin to kick in.

6

THE STRESS–PROCRASTINATION CONTINUUM

When we procrastinate, we literally create our own stress. The activities we avoid seem to grow larger and larger, finally appearing more difficult and more threatening than they really are.

Yet an opportunity lies hidden in procrastination. When we take action on the activities we have been avoiding, we feel immediate relief and energy to move ahead with all the activities in our lives. It is a classic example of a good stress that appears to be bad until we act upon it. At that point, we experience the relief, energy, and other unexpected benefits that come when good stress is released.

Not all procrastination is the same. If you are stalling about cleaning the gutters, that is obviously not the same as avoiding a conversation with your spouse to work out the details of your separation.

There are different kinds of procrastination, and they have different effects on the way we sense and process stress. Let's take a closer look.

Cumulative Procrastination

The habit of letting routine small tasks pile up is one of the most common forms of stress-producing procrastination. People who suffer from it are so enmeshed in the pattern, they don't often recognize it as the stressor it has become in day-to-day life.

Although cumulative procrastination can strike at home, its symptoms are easiest to see on the job, a setting where most of us have to complete many low-level tasks every day. When people have become victims to it, their desks are piled high with message slips, memos and unopened mail. Often, the clutter has spilled onto windowsills, empty chairs, and the floor. Computer monitors are papered thick with reminders scribbled on Post-it notes.

Then, when habitual cumulative procrastinators are required to handle a new task, they don't handle it on the spot. Instead, they just add it to the quagmire of other uncompleted tasks, intending to do it later. Their work has become a large, undifferentiated morass. Often, the man or woman who has become a victim to this pattern is highly stressed. Each new duty to perform is perceived as a new stimulus that triggers a reaction of fight or flight.

Workers who have *not* fallen victim to the cumulative-procrastination trap are also easy to spot. (In most organizations, they really stand out because there are so few of them.) When they leave work at the end of each day, their desks are free of clutter. Some of them actually live by the ancient time-management rule Touch any piece of paper only once.

When we watch these nonprocrastinators at work, their secret becomes clear. They have simply cultivated the habit of completing minor tasks immediately. When that is not possible because they are performing another task, they handle the new task as soon as they reasonably can.

Of course, cumulative procrastination does not strike us only on the job. When it attacks domestic life, the sufferer's home becomes cluttered. Routine maintenance activities such as shopping, cleaning, or taking out the garbage are handled in a catch-as-catch-can way. Of course, this pattern can make home life unnecessarily tense.

Cumulative procrastination is especially likely to gain hold over nonessential personal activities. A cumulative procrastinator, for example, might agree to act as head of a committee in his town but never quite gets started. All commitments get delayed and delayed as the stress builds.

Once cumulative procrastination has gained control over us, it can be hard to stop. But it really can be tackled. And once that is accomplished, the feelings of competence that follow are often gratifying enough to keep the problem away for good. The key is usually getting started.

Attack the symptoms head-on. If your office is piled with papers, you can go into your office one Saturday morning for a clutter-busting blitz. Simply pick up one pile of papers at a time and process it. The TRAF approach explained by organizational expert Stephanie Winston can be highly effective in this process: You pick up one piece of paper at a time and either Toss it, Refer it to someone else, Act on it at once, or File it. Or if you've been avoiding a time-consuming nonwork activity (the church committee, school event), break the deadlock decisively by making a mailing or asking a few friends to join you on the committee. Simply take the first step that will get you started.

Establish routines to handle maintenance tasks automatically. After you have attacked the problem directly, routines can help keep it at bay. After you have reduced the clutter in your office or your home, for example, you can empty your entire in box every day at eleven A.M. and process its contents instead of adding them to the piles that are already on your desk. The feelings of efficacy that result from such new habits are usually more pleasurable than old patterns of avoidance. Once you get started, you feel more and more motivated to keep going.

Create a long-range schedule for tasks you have been avoiding. If you've been letting a number of home-maintenance projects pile up, for example, decide that next weekend you will call a painter, look through paint swatches, and get an estimate. The weekend after that, you will remove the dented, nonworking lighting along your driveway and install new fixtures. A schedule is a potent tool for chasing stress away. Just mark everything down.

Conflict-Avoidance Procrastination

Delaying conflict with other people is a pattern of procrastination that's even more stressful than cumulative procrastination.

Often, the situations we avoid are relatively inconsequential, such as telling your teenager she cannot go to an unsupervised party with her friends next Saturday. At other times, the conflicts we're avoiding promise to be more serious, such as telling your boss his pet project won't be completed on deadline or calling the Internal Revenue Service to negotiate a schedule for paying taxes that are past due.

When we avoid conflict, we experience procrastination's full power to make problems appear larger and more threatening than they really are. Even worse, our pattern of avoidance can become habitual. Whenever we face a problem that promises disagreement, we avoid it. As with cumulative-procrastination stress, issues pile up and become a paralyzing force that can keep us immobilized in a state of chronic bad stress.

(We see conflict-avoidance-procrastination stress in many areas of our lives. When your son comes home and says he is being picked on by a tough older kid on the school playground, you can see how that bully is utilizing your son's natural tendency to avoid conflict to throw him into a pitiable state of anxiety. Sadly, this manipulative pattern does not disappear once our school years are completed. It persists in many areas of adult lives through bullying bosses, manipulative colleagues, and more.)

One danger of conflict-avoidance-procrastination stress is that it tends to disguise itself as something else in the mind of the sufferer. Some parents avoid confronting their children about drinking, drugs, or important issues where they should intervene, telling themselves they are being "sensitive" and "respectful of privacy" in their parenting role. Still other people assure themselves that when they submit to the control of self-proclaimed authority figures (domineering bosses, kids' over-bearing teachers, authoritarians of all kinds), they are really behaving with appropriate respect before "experts" who know more than they do.

Over time, conflict-avoidance-procrastination stress can become chronic, leading to personal feelings of powerlessness. Yet there are ways to break free of its hold.

Do a "worst-case scenario" of conflicts you are avoiding. What is the worst thing that could happen when you tell your employee that you are about to document his poor attendance in a memo to his personnel file, or if you confront your hot-headed supervisor and tell him your budget is about to be late? Such confrontations, while disquieting, generally yield reassuring answers. If you confront that worker, his performance won't get any worse because it couldn't. He might actually improve. If you tell your boss that your budget will be late, you will probably be able to work out a revised schedule to complete it.

Ask for feedback from a trustworthy and impartial mentor. Simply describe your problem to someone whom you completely trust: your spouse, an old friend, a college professor, a member of the clergy at your place of worship. Describe the parameters of the situation (your kid's science teacher has a demeaning tone that undermines the students' self-esteem and you have to confront him about it; you need to confront your neighbor about excessive noise) and ask for feedback. How serious does the problem appear to your mentor? What advice can he or she offer about how to proceed?

Recall similar conflicts in the past to find motivation to act decisively now. What happened when you confronted a demeaning colleague last year, when you contested a traffic ticket in court, or when you told a relative you did not want to invest money in his harebrained moneymaking scheme? Chances are that the problem was more easily resolved than you expected. By reviewing the outcomes of past conflicts, you put your current one in context and gain the courage to face the problem down.

Discomfort Procrastination

Discomfort procrastination is a particularly insidious form of stress-induced postponement which, like the other forms described above, is often invisible to its victim. It gains power over us through its power to delude us about the real reasons we are putting things off.

In a very common example, a man (or a woman) decides to start a program of exercise. He joins a health club, buys appropriate exercise clothing, and then never starts. (Ready, set, wait!) He tells himself he doesn't like to exercise, but that is probably not the problem at all. He is really avoiding the discomfort that will occur when he enters a new, unfamiliar situation.

- He will not know where the lockers are.
- He might look laughable in his new exercise clothing.
- The exercises might be too difficult or even painful.
- He will have to meet new people, who might already be chummy and see him as an intrusion.

So what he is immediately avoiding is not exercise (though that might be part of the problem), but the discomfort of entering into a new situation.

In another common scenario, a woman (or man) decides to quit her fast-paced corporate job, step back, and start a new career in teaching. She contacts her state board of education, fills out the papers, but never sends them in. (Ready, set, wait! again) In her mind she's obsessing about a vague scenario.

⯈ Her relatives, friends, and neighbors will think she is a failure.

⯈ She will no longer get invited to parties with her former friends.

⯈ She will make so little money that she will have to drive around in a shabby old car.

And on it goes. Again the sufferer is not avoiding the change she is contemplating per se, but succumbing to fears about the discomfort that will accompany changes.

Remedies for Discomfort Procrastination

There is a good side to discomfort procrastination. Once the sufferer realizes he or she has become a victim to it, there are often simple cures.

Break down the problem you are facing into two parts. Part one is the issue you are avoiding (starting to exercise, changing a career). Part two is the discomfort that accompanies it. Once you have parsed the problem in this way, you are able to attack the discomfort as a problem separate from the rest. On the morning you are visiting the health club for your first workout, you can tell yourself, "Okay, this is new territory and I'm going to feel gawkish. But that's unimportant in light of the importance of getting back in shape."

Test the waters. If you're contemplating a career change that might entail a reduction in income, work out a budget and pin down the specifics. Or if you are afraid about how friends in your community might react to the news of the change you've made, invite one of them to lunch ahead of time to discuss the change you are contemplating. In all likelihood, a friend will be pleased to hear you are contemplating a career change that will bring you greater happiness. Your fears will probably disappear.

Make a provisional start. If you're going to the YMCA to start exercising, call ahead to arrange a tour so you can eliminate uncertainties about the physical layout, where you should go, etc. Ask for a training session on the equipment you'll use. When the first day of your actual workout regimen begins, make it a "dry run" in which you'll drive to the facility, go in, find a locker, visit the area you'll be using (the pool, weight room, etc.), and enjoy a light workout of fifteen to thirty minutes at most. Then leave and resume your day. With the sources of uncertainty and discomfort diminished, your next visit can be your first "real" workout. Because you have removed the sources of discomfort procrastination, you are free to start your exercise routine for real, and unencumbered by stress.

7

DISCOVERING GOOD STRESS'S POWER TO BUILD A MORE REWARDING CAREER

Nobody enjoys career dissatisfaction. Yet if we arm ourselves with the right knowledge and understanding, our career "rumblings" and "frictions" usually turn out to be good stresses in disguise. If we can heed the messages they bring us and take action, we move to new levels of career satisfaction and success.

Career dissatisfaction and stress can strike us at different career stages, for seemingly different reasons.

- A young woman feels suddenly unsure about the career she has chosen. Yes, she just earned a college degree in communications. But now that she's two months into her first job as a production assistant for a television station, she's not so sure she made the right career choice. She's not applying the skills and knowledge she learned in college. Each day new situations arise that she doesn't know how to handle. She's hit a period of unexpected career stress.

- Late in his career, a marketing executive feels suddenly unsettled about the work he has been doing for two decades. All at once it doesn't seem to "mean anything." He begins to feel odd impulses he's never felt before. One day he's thinking about quitting his job and becoming a teacher. The next, about taking the money he's saved so he can buy a sailboat and cruise around the Caribbean, watching sunsets. And on the job his attitude has suddenly changed. The tasks he used to relish have seem monotonous. Some days he doesn't return phone calls. All these changes make him worry. Is the whole house of cards, the career he's worked so hard to build, about to come raining down around him?

Getting to the Roots of Career Dissatisfaction

The two people described above are experiencing career dissatisfaction at the opposite poles of working life. One is at the start of a career, the other in the late stages. On the surface their situations would appear to be completely different. Yet that is probably not the case. Nina H. Frost, a career counselor with New York's Vocare Group and one of the authors of *Soul Mapping: An Imaginative Way to Self-Discovery*, believes that these two people are probably experiencing their career stresses for very similar reasons.

"Learning is the factor that underlies career satisfaction," Frost says. "When we are learning in the right kind of way, we usually feel like we belong in our work. When learning is not there, or when we experience frictions and uncertainties surrounding it, that's when we begin to think 'I've outgrown my job' or 'Did I make the right career choice?'"

According to Frost, our career satisfaction depends on lifelong learning. To be satisfied in our work, we need to feel that our jobs "pull something out of us," that we are being stretched and grown by our work. When that is not happening, the stresses we feel represent positive clues that we need to make changes. Let's take a closer look.

The Four Quadrants of Career Growth

Frost has determined that during our years of working, we pass through four career quadrants that are closely related to our need to learn and grow.

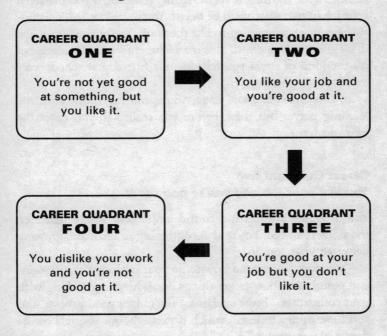

CAREER QUADRANT ONE

You're not yet good at something, but you like it.

CAREER QUADRANT TWO

You like your job and you're good at it.

CAREER QUADRANT FOUR

You dislike your work and you're not good at it.

CAREER QUADRANT THREE

You're good at your job but you don't like it.

Career Quadrant One:
You're not yet good at something but you like it.

A lot of stress is present during this early career phase, but it is positive stress that arises when we undergo a lot of personal growth quickly. This is the quadrant where the young woman we described at the start of this chapter finds herself. She's under a lot of stress. Each day thrusts her into new situations that make her wonder whether she has what it takes to make it in her chosen field. Yet it is a stimulating and exciting phase.

"This is what the Zen thinkers call a 'Beginner's Mind,'" Frost explains. "You feel as though you don't know anything about what you are doing. You're all nerves and adrenaline. You haven't mastered the tasks fully, you don't understand the politics of your company, you might not even know where the bathroom is. But all the learning is very exciting. After all, if you mastered your job in two days, you'd be bored. You've been hired, presumably, because you're going to like the work. You're going to shape it, it's going to shape you. This is an inherently stressful stage, but it's the kind of stress you felt on your first day at school, very exciting."

In this first-quadrant stage, you're moving quickly up the learning curve. But then, before you realize it, you enter the next quadrant.

Career Quadrant Two:
You like your job and you're good at it.

You now feel assured and confident because you've mastered the skills you need. You're also continuing to learn and growing better at what you do.

"You now understand how to do your job, what the customs and politics are, how to get things done, how to get along with your compadres," Frost explains. "You're in a good groove. You still have things to learn, which is exciting, but you feel confident and competent."

This is a very happy stage. But troubles lie ahead. "Nobody tells you that this phase won't last twenty years," Frost explains. "Even though this is a stress-free point in your life, you unfortunately can't stay there."

It is at this point in our careers that we really need to be thinking about our next career activities. We can't stay on this plateau forever. Yet because we feel comfortable where we are, we rarely look ahead.

At some point, however, change intrudes. Our need to learn and grow makes itself felt as we move on to the next career quadrant.

Career Quadrant Three:
You're Good at Your Job but You Don't Like It.

This is where career discontents begin to creep in. People at this stage report they are beginning to "outgrow" their careers or that they are looking for "something more." Some people look outside their companies at other companies or at their contemporaries for the first time in years, and they worry that life is passing them by.

"It can take months or years to arrive at this phase," Frost explains. "You're actually becoming a victim of your own skills and competence. The newness is gone. You're not learning and you often feel like you're just going through the motions."

At this phase, people often make changes in their careers; sometimes the *wrong* changes. They start to believe that their dissatisfactions are tied to the organization where they work and they miss the deeper messages that their stress might contain. A lawyer might blame her discontent on the firm where she is a partner. An auto service manager might leave Honda to work for Ford.

"At times, catapulting yourself into something new might be called for," Frost explains. "But it can be even more important to consider your job and your career in a different way. Thinking again of learning, you might ask what happened to the newness and the excitement and stimulation you felt early in your career. How can you find ways to regain it now? Sometimes doing so is a matter of expanding your role, perhaps switching sectors or departments so you can keep on growing."

Making change in just this way is talked about more and more today, often called "career redeployment" or "recareering." It involves taking critical action to keep a career growing.

If we do not take the right steps to reinvent our careers at this stage, we enter into the fourth and most disruptive career quadrant.

Career Quadrant Four:
You dislike your work and you're not good at it.

Here we find the marketing executive we met at the beginning of this chapter. Not only is he miserable in his job, he is beginning to make some serious mistakes. If the job burnout he feels at this stage is especially acute, he may not even be too concerned that is happening.

"At this stage you become very bad at something," Frost explains, "even though, of course, you are *very* good at it when you want to be."

Frost explains that many executives who have been fired often tell her troubling stories about the mistakes and miscalculations they made in this career phase. "After they have voiced all the horror and the shock and the outrage about being fired, they eventually have a little sheepish moment when they say, 'Well, I did kind of have something to do with the fact that I'm no longer there. I guess I did engineer my own demise.' Yet it is often true that without that 'demise,' they would never have taken healthy steps toward a new life."

Many executives also make career miscalculations and mistakes at this phase, often starting ill-advised new businesses that don't last too long or leaving in anger to take the wrong jobs.

Curiously the best resolution to the problems that arise in this quadrant is often to loop back to a new career situation that closely resembles those of the first quadrant.

In other words, when we find ourselves in acute burnout, it is a usable sign that we need to again put ourselves into a situation that demands intense learning and growth, perhaps by starting your own company or taking a new position that makes radical new demands on you. The alternative is to remain bored and stuck.

It takes a lot of courage to make this transition by leaving the security of a longstanding career and put yourself in the path of change. "Many people invent all kinds of reasons why they cannot make the very move they know is required," Frost states. "They say they can't afford the financial risk, or that people wouldn't understand why they have given up security and tried something new and risky. In such cases, it can be quite helpful to make the big changes in a series of small, exploratory steps. You can keep one foot in the old world while testing the new."

The real question at this point is whether it is riskier to try something new, offering potential rewards, than to remain in a job or career that has already become destabilized and dangerous. Given Frost's explanation of these quadrants, it seems that taking the apparently riskier path (heeding the messages that stress brings and making essential changes) may actually be the safest route of all.

Exercise

Take a look at where you are in your career.

LOOK at the career quadrant chart on page 59 and ask some pointed questions.

- ◗ Which quadrant are you in now?
- ◗ How do you know? What symptoms, exactly, led you to place yourself there?
- ◗ What are you learning in your current phase? Does it satisfy your need to grow in your career?
- ◗ Looking ahead to the next quadrant, what issues and concerns should you start to think about today?
- ◗ If you are already experiencing severe career stress (which is most likely to occur in quadrants three or four), what kind of career redefinition can you engage in now so you can begin a new growth phase in your work?

8

USING GOOD STRESS
TO SOLVE PROBLEMS

Most of us expend time and mental energy "dealing with" problems. Yet how effective are our efforts? How often do we unlock the good stress in the problems we're facing and make something positive out of them?

At any given time, we might be "dealing with" many different issues, including:

- Grief over the loss of a loved one or friend
- Concern about a son's or daughter's social issues
- Anger about conflicts on the job
- Worry about health-related concerns
- Struggles to break habits such as eating too much, drinking, or smoking
- Financial issues such as saving for retirement

When we look at a list as varied as that, we realize that "dealing with," a concept most people think they understand is not really one process at all, but a catchphrase that bundles together worry, grief, planning, behavior modification and many more processes too.

In fact, if you stop to examine your overall success with the problems you're facing, you may be in for quite a surprise. While you have been "dealing with" problems, you have not eliminated any of them or made progress on them.

A Quick Test of Your Problem-Solving Skills

Try this simple three-step test to see how effective you are at problem-solving:

First, list the three or four major issues you are "dealing with" today.

Second, make a list of three or four issues you were "dealing with" one year ago.

Third, to the best of your ability, create the same list for two years ago, three years ago, and five.

Compare all these lists. If they are essentially the same, if the biggest problems remain unsolved, you may not be really "dealing with" difficulties at all but obsessing about them and actually letting them add to your sensations of chronic stress.

Why Some Problems Refuse to Go Away

Certain problems are serious and can't be made to go away too quickly. Grief, marital frictions, chronic illnesses, and vocational problems all require time. But many of us are adding to our stress by deluding ourselves that we are solving problems, when less productive processes are really at work.

▶ We're pretending we want to eliminate a particular problem, but down deep we do not want to eradicate it at all. It might even have become part of our self-definition.

▶ We're beating ourselves up about a problem so we can enjoy a sense of self-pity about it. That self-coddling

would disappear if we processed the problem and
moved on with our lives.

▶ We're procrastinating about problems we *could* control
if we ever got started. But we delay.

▶ We're so worried about the negative consequences of
taking action that we think it's safer to remain stuck
and go on living in undifferentiated stress.

These are some reasons that people become stuck and stressed
about chronic problems. Year after year, they "need to lose fifteen
pounds" or "get their finances in order" or "sell this old house and
move." They believe they're dealing with these issues, but they
are really treading water, staying stuck in one place.

Converting Problems to Plans

If you find you've been processing the same problems for too
long instead of moving ahead, an effective first corrective step
is to invest a little time analyzing the words you have chosen to
describe your problem to friends, family members, and yourself.
Although analyzing language has become a staple of "pop-
psych" books in recent years, there is some validity to the exercise. The language you've chosen to describe the issues you are
grappling with can offer clues to self-defeating behaviors. Here
are two common discoveries that result from this exercise.

You find you are defeating yourself with unrealistic expectations. If you're in the habit of saying or thinking "I need to lose
thirty pounds and get into really great shape," for example, you
have set out intimidating tasks for yourself and you probably
will never find the initiative to get started. ("Why even try
when I'm so overweight and out of shape?")

You realize you have not defined the problem clearly enough
to start working on it. If you've been saying "I've got to find
another job," you have only created an unfocused statement of

the issue that prevents you from envisioning the specific steps that will give you the "traction" to move ahead.

The next step is to pin things down in new language that is not self-defeating and is specific enough to be actionable.

If you've been saying "I need to lose thirty pounds and get into great shape," for example, you would do well to break that amorphous statement down into a plan that might include steps like these:

- Meet with my physician for a physical and some advice before beginning a program of dieting and exercise.
- Visit four exercise facilities near where I live and select the place I'd like to start my workouts.
- Go to a library or bookstore and bring home four new cookbooks on interesting, flavorful low-fat cooking that will satisfy my interest in eating well as I start to lose weight.
- Stop thinking about how much weight I want to lose and start to engage in some positive new behaviors that will lead to a healthier lifestyle.

Or if you've been saying, "I've got to find another job," break things down into steps like these:

- Join my industry association to network and assure that I am current with the latest trends.
- Revitalize my professional network by calling two former contacts and colleagues each week to reestablish contact with them.
- Familiarize myself with the wide range of new Internet career resources.
- Show my résumé next week to some members of my network for their comments and suggestions.

There is one additional step to take in this planning phase too. That is to schedule when and how you will take the steps you plan, using actual dates and times you write into your date book, digital device, calendar, or whatever tracking system you use to manage your time.

In this way, problems become plans you can act upon. And when they do, you experience the sensation of relief that comes when good stress is released by taking positive action.

Suppose You Still Can't Get Moving?

What happens if you take the steps suggested above (setting reasonable expectations and making the problem clear) and you still cannot get started in processing your plans? If that happens, the next step is to confront a rather difficult question: Do I really want to solve this problem?

That question can be hard to answer. Yet the answers it demands can help uncover inner hesitations that are holding you back.

Some psychologists have even suggested that when we are unable to move ahead on problems we feel we should be addressing, we should literally give up on them, cross them right off the mental to-do list of the issues we are involved with in our lives. We should actively decide *not* to diet, *not* to exercise, *not* to engage in difficult conversations with our children about drugs. At this point of surrender, we often encounter an "inner voice" that provides new insights into what is holding us back.

If you find yourself thinking, for example, "I cannot give up on losing weight *because I would disappoint my friends and parents,*" you might decide that your efforts to lose weight would be more successful if you envisioned personal rewards or dieting, not rewards for other people. Of if you think, "I cannot stop monitoring my cholesterol level—*my children need me to be around for another twenty years*," you have bumped into a new impetus to solve problems energetically and move ahead.

Another highly effective way to break inertia is to simply take action in one very small part of a plan you have created to address your problem. For example, you can call a friend and say, "I need to start exercising but don't know how. Do you have any suggestions?" Or if you need to tune up the technical skills you need at work before starting a job hunt, enroll in a class or simply search for training resources on the Internet.

Taking even a very small, nonthreatening step toward your goal is often all that is required to establish momentum to move ahead.

9

RESOLVE CONFLICTS
WITH GOOD STRESS

Paul and Susan's marriage was in trouble. From his side of the relationship, Paul knew that he and his wife were no longer spending enough time together or communicating well. From her vantage point, Susan felt that Paul had withdrawn from her emotionally and physically. Yet they had both decided not to discuss the question. Paul was worried that if they started talking, he and Susan would get divorced and he would lose the comfort of his home and his stable domestic routines. Susan feared that if she initiated a discussion, she would drive Paul even further away and lose still more of the intimacy she wanted. They were living every day in a state of ongoing stress.

Paul and Susan are fictional characters, but problems like theirs are familiar to marriage counselors and psychotherapists. They represent two people who stand frozen between two contradictory goals at the same time. Paul wants to discuss his dissatisfaction with Susan, but he also wants to preserve a comfortable domestic life. If he pursues either goal whole-heartedly, he believes he must give up its counterpart goal on the other side. Susan finds herself in a similar predicament. She wants more intimacy from Paul, but if she confronts him about it, she just might drive him further into hiding. Like many people in conflict, they choose not to act and go on living in a state of chronic tension and stress.

We have all experienced this kind of stress at some point in our lives. Sometimes the pattern of conflict has been with us so long, we forget it is there. We are aware only of the unhappiness and stress it brings.

You are familiar with conflict-based stress if you have been in stalemates like these:

⟩ You felt completely burned out in your job, but you were only five years from retirement. You needed to keep working to receive your full pension. So you put up with the stress until you reached age sixty-five.

⟩ You didn't want to marry your college boyfriend, but you didn't want to lose the relationship either. So you stuck it out and remained in an unsatisfying, conflicted relationship until you both graduated and went your separate ways.

⟩ You were paying a great deal of money to an extended-care facility every month to care for your mother, but at the same time you felt pressure to move your growing family out of your apartment into a house. As home prices spiraled upward, you felt a gnawing fear that you would never be able to afford the house you dreamed of.

Living in conflict brings on all the negative effects of chronic stress. It erodes our relationships, lowers our self-esteem, and harms our health. For some people, it can lead to alcohol abuse and other self-destructive behaviors. Yet even when we realize that we are facing conflict and understand that we need to decide how to end it, it is not always so easy to move forward. Like deer who stand frozen in the path of an oncoming car, we stay where we are, unable to move to the right or the left.

By refusing to act, we sometimes think we are protecting ourselves. ("Nothing bad will happen to me if I just hide here.") Yet inaction is really action. By refusing to act, we are actually making a hidden decision that can be very destructive. Over time, our "nondecisions" cause stress to snowball, making our problems bigger, more threatening, and harder to solve.

Using ICEPTA to Break Conflict Stress

I urge you to follow the steps of the ICEPTA process, which I designed to help people discover and resolve conflicts in their lives. ICEPTA is an acronym that stands for Identify, Clarify, Explore, Plan, Take action, and Adapt.

Let's take a closer look at putting each step of this process to work.

Identify Areas of Conflict in Your Life

As you read this chapter, it has probably become obvious to you that some of the stresses you discovered in your Personal Stress Inventory are conflict based. Perhaps you and your former spouse squabble about when and where your children will spend their time. Or you dislike your job and would like to start your own company but don't want to give up the security of a steady paycheck.

At other times, conflict will be a less obvious cause of stress. You will have to discover that it is there. For this reason, it is a good idea to review the list of acutely stressful situations that resulted from the Personal Stress Inventory. Look at those issues singly and try to decide which of them might involve conflict that you have not recognized. Perhaps you responded that "shopping for food and personal items" was highly stressful but did not realize when you completed the Personal Stress Inventory that the real cause of that stress was conflict with your spouse over domestic routines. Or maybe you responded that you found "office politics" highly stressful but didn't pinpoint the fact that you and one colleague are competing for the next available promotion.

Recognizing that we are facing conflict is the first step toward resolving it. It is not unlike the first step of the 12-step recovery programs, which is to *admit* that you have a problem.

Clarify the Conflict

The next step is to clarify the nature of your stress by describing it as simply as you can. In practical terms, this means boiling the conflict down to its essential elements so you can understand where you can start working to resolve it.

For some conflicts, this clarification can be simple. ("My car requires constant repairs and I need to buy a new one, but I am already carrying too much debt to afford one.") When you are describing more complex conflicts, you will probably end up with a list of different issues that are contributing to the overall stress.

As an example, let's examine a conflict mentioned moments ago: Imagine that you and your former spouse are squabbling about when and where your children will spend their time during the week and on weekends. A description of the stressful aspects of this conflict might include the following:

- ▶ Weekend routines with your kids were the most pleasant aspect of your former marriage and you're grieving because those patterns are now lost.
- ▶ You and your former spouse practice different religions and you object to having your kids attend services at his or her place of worship.
- ▶ Your former spouse has remarried and you fear that your kids will begin to like this "other" mom or dad more than they like you.
- ▶ You feel that your former in-laws spoil your children and you don't want them around your kids when you are not there.

As you analyze conflict-based stresses in this way, the causes of conflict come suddenly into sharper focus. Instead of a hazy, undifferentiated area of stress in your life ("my relationship with my former husband"), you are dealing with some specific issues ("I feel that he spends too much money on our kids as a way to win their favor").

The more you can boil conflict down to specifics, the more you equip yourself to break its hold on your life.

Explore Possible Solutions

In the E step in the process, it is time to explore ways to resolve the conflict you have identified. As you completed the C step, you might have glimpsed some of the options available to you. Yet before you fix on just what your next step will be, it is a good idea to obtain objective advice and help. Some appropriate actions might be to:

> ❯ Meet with a trustworthy mentor who can offer objective advice. Depending on the nature of the conflict you are facing, this person might be a close friend, a minister or clergy person, a psychotherapist, a lawyer, or an accountant. Describe the conflict you are facing and ask for advice and ideas.
>
> ❯ Gather information on the kind of conflict you are facing by reading books and articles, conducting Internet searches, etc.
>
> ❯ Attend a meeting of a support group or other organization made up of people who have faced conflicts similar to yours.

At this point, you are exploring your options. The more ideas you can gather, the better equipped you become to pick an appropriate course of action to move you out of your conflict.

Plan What Steps You Will Take

Clarifying the nature of your conflict and exploring possible solutions are only a prelude to conflict resolution. The next step is to plot out the specific steps you will take to resolve the issues you have identified. This means being quite specific.

- Instead of obsessing about your inability to afford a new car, you will meet with your accountant to review your finances and find a way to better manage your debt.
- Instead of having constant skirmishes with your siblings about the kind of care you are providing for your dad, you will all meet with an eldercare consultant/specialist to select appropriate options.
- Instead of fretting about your inability to get out of a conflict-laden job, you will plan to attend a job fair, talk to prospective new employers, and take courses to build your technical skill if necessary.

Interesting to note, it is sometimes possible to resolve conflict at this step by realizing that you are powerless to resolve the conflict you are confronting. If you are worried that your in-laws will spoil your kids with expensive gifts and excursions, you might realize that there is really nothing you can do about it. It is a situation out of your control. What you *can* do to resolve the stress, however, is adjust your own reaction to it by taking a new perspective or attitude. You can't keep your kids away from your mother-in-law and father-in-law, but you can decide the problem is not important enough to cause the emotional turmoil and distress you have allowed it to exert over you. By making a considered decision not to act, you have actually taken steps to control your stress.

Take Action in the Area of Conflict

The T step of the ICEPTA process may seem odd and unnec-
essary. After all, you have conceptualized your stressful problem, explored possible solutions, and planned what you will do.
But unless you take those intentions and act on them, you are
certain to remain stalled. You have caught yourself in a trap of
constantly *preparing* and never *doing*. It's a kind of "ready, aim .
. . aim . . . aim" pattern that creates a false, immobilizing illu-
sion that you are processing a conflict when in fact you are not.

Your calendar or appointment book can be your best tool in
breaking any deadlocks. Instead of deciding you will make an
appointment "someday" with your former spouse to discuss
three or four issues you've pinpointed about your parenting
duties, you call and make an appointment for *next Saturday*.
Instead of planning to meet with a financial consultant "when
you can," you take out your calendar and call to make an
appointment for *next week*.

Without action-taking, conflict lingers and the stress it
brings gets worse.

Adapt and Adjust

If your approach to dealing with conflict is to issue ultimatums
and make rigid demands, you are almost certainly condemning
yourself to prolong the conflict-based situation that is making
your life stressful. The best approach is usually to adopt a
problem-solving, cooperative approach instead.

If you want to escape from an unpleasant job without losing
all your benefits, present that problem to a company official in
human resources and be open to his or her suggestion instead
of saying, "Tell me how I can get out of here today and keep all
my benefits." Often, a compromise or provisional resolution to
your problem is available if you are flexible enough to accept it.

If your husband loves your kids' school and you think it is doing a bad job of educating them, present your points and listen to his arguments. Chances are a compromise or joint solution can be worked out once you get into the specifics. (You think the math program at the school is lacking, your spouse feels the good social climate outweighs that deficiency; perhaps you can solve the conflict by enrolling your kids in an after-school math program to bolster that area of weak instruction.) A cooperative attitude will produce better results than a confrontational one. ("The kids' school stinks, yet you insist on keeping them there.")

By remaining flexible and adaptive, you equip yourself to move flexibly around areas of conflict in your life instead of allowing them to keep you mired in friction and stress.

Exercise

**Use ICEPTA to identify a conflict and plan
your solution to it.**

TAKE one area of conflict in your life and create a tentative
plan for how you would move it forward through the ICEP-
TA steps, finally causing it to be resolved. For example, you
might:

▶ Identify the problem: You run a retail operation
with a partner and are in constant disagreement
about how he fulfills his end of the agreement.

▶ Clarify the problem: He spends the company
resources without your prior permission, in ways
you see as wasteful.

▶ Explore possible solutions: You could meet with
two trusted mentors (your brother, a management
professor you studied with in college) and ask
their advice on resolving the conflict. You could
also contact the Service Corps of Retired
Executives (an organization of retired business-
people who offer free counseling to small businesses) and ask to speak with a counselor who
can offer you advice on resolving issues related to
partnerships.

▶ Plan by identifying three or four points of friction
you need to discuss with your partner.

▶ Take action by scheduling a meeting.

▶ Adapt and adjust by presenting your concerns,
allowing your partner to present his, and deciding
whether you can create a joint decision-making
process that will allow you both to agree upon
expenditures before they are made.

If you apply this imaginary application of ICEPTA to a problem you are facing, you will engage in a mental "workout" that will tell you that conflict is a condition that appears to be insoluble and chronic but which responds to action-taking.

10

How Good Stress Can
Make Our Closest
Relationships Stronger

Along with all the good feelings, it's natural to feel some tension in our love relationships. We often find those stresses bad. After all, our closest relationships are supposed to be a source of pleasure. Yet instead of immediately classifying areas of interpersonal friction as threatening or bad, another path is available to us. We can explore whether the stressful areas in our relationships are calling our attention to issues that need our attention if we are to grow closer to our partners.

We all experience stresses in our marriages and closest relationships. After all, how could two complex human beings come together as spouses, partners, or intimate friends without friction? It would be irrational to expect anything else.

Yet illogical or not, many of us jump to the conclusion that something is terribly wrong when our love relationships are not completely placid and stress free. If we encounter an area of friction, we are quick to classify it as bad stress that has the potential to destabilize the relationship.

We know we've touched such threatening "hot spots" when we find ourselves making statements like these:

- "My wife became nearly hysterical last year when I said we ought to meet with a lawyer to prepare our wills. I can't get up the nerve to mention it again."
- "I can't even talk to my boyfriend about how much his brothers take advantage of him. I'm only trying to pro-

tect him, but when I speak up he gets angry because I'm criticizing his kin."

▶ "Sometimes I feel like I just can't count on my best friend. When she calls and really needs to talk about something, I put aside everything and make the time for her. When the situation is reversed and I need to talk, she's suddenly too busy. I'm always giving more than she is."

Avoiding Avoidance

When we encounter such interpersonal frictions, the most natural tendency is to look the other way. We believe that if we can simply skirt that ticklish area or uncomfortable topic, we will enjoy a more placid and stress-free relationship. Or we adopt a "not-today" policy, hoping the problem will resolve itself on its own.

In some cases, this avoidance does work, allowing us to tiptoe around a conflict temporarily and keep the peace. In other instances, however, avoiding problems only makes problems dormant for a time until they erupt, doing more serious damage.

▶ The man who can't discuss the issue of estate planning with his wife finally becomes so frustrated that he visits a lawyer by himself to draft their wills. When he tells his wife what he has done, she feels betrayed and deeply hurt. What was a simple communication problem has now caused a major calamity in the relationship.

▶ The woman who feels resentment toward her boyfriend's brothers bottles up her anger for as long as possible. But then, at a family party, the pressure becomes too much to bear and she starts a major argument that *really* serves to destabilize the relationship.

▶ The woman who feels she can't count on her best friend retaliates by starting to say she is unavailable when her friend calls to chat. Within a year, this behavior puts an end to her most important friendship.

Good Stresses Masquerading as Bad

This chapter opened with the statement that many stresses in love relationships are actually positive, directing our attention to issues that need to be solved before we can grow closer to our loved ones. Let's take a closer look.

Good Stress Opportunity #1:
Frictions Caused by Different Communication Styles

We all know that miscommunication is a leading cause of interpersonal friction. Yet we might not be aware of a small wrinkle in that principle: Different communication *styles* cause a lot of friction too, sometimes making essentially good relationships appear troubled.

A story reported in the book *Where Do I Go from Here?* by Dr. Kenneth Ruge provides a revealing example of the stress and potential damage that can result when two people simply communicate in different ways.

Dr. Ruge, a psychotherapist and marriage counselor, had been visited by a married couple who were experiencing a lot of friction in their relationship. The more they described the issues that were upsetting them, the clearer it became to them that they were experiencing the stress that can be caused by differing communication styles.

The woman came from a family with a Mediterranean background. As a group, they were very ebullient in their communications style—loud and quick to take issue with one another.

The man came from a family with its roots in northern Europe. They were a taciturn group of people who, by and large, never raised their voices unless something truly catastrophic was taking place. After their wedding, these communications styles collided. When voicing opinions, the woman would be very vocal and emphatic; her husband couldn't understand why his wife was "angry" at him. The woman, from her point of view, couldn't understand why her husband was holding so much in, not communicating, and becoming "withdrawn."

Both partners were "bottling up" the problem and worrying about the stability of their marriage. Yet when Dr. Ruge, an objective observer, pointed out that they were not really arguing but experiencing conflicting communications styles, the gray clouds began to dissipate.

By having the courage to explore the roots of the stresses they felt instead of evading the issue, they were able to confront deep-seated issues that might have actually destabilized their marriage over time. With the problem behind them, they were actually able to laugh about it and grow closer.

Good Stress Opportunity #2:
Unspoken Expectations

Unvoiced expectations can function as still another hot spot in relationships. If left unvoiced over time, they threaten to destabilize even the strongest relationships. Consider these common examples:

Unspoken desires about having children. Problems often arise when a husband or wife enters into a marriage with a strong-but-unspoken desire to have children—or *not* to have children. Perhaps some masking behavior has taken place: one partner feared his partner would not have wanted to get married if he or she openly stated a position on the subject. At some point, it becomes an issue that cannot be avoided any longer.

Differing expectations about the parameters of a relation-

ship. Your best friend calls and, for the first time, complains openly about her husband's drinking. You are shocked and stressed at first because you thought that your relationship was too casual to include such sensitive issues. She is pushing back the boundaries, striving to make your relationship more intimate than before. Your immediate impulse might be to reject this sudden overture. ("We're not such close friends.") But you might also decide to respond in kind by introducing a sensitive topic of your own, effectively agreeing to deepen your friendship. It is one of those turning points that can either strengthen friendships or make them sour.

Silent long-term plans. Perhaps your husband always thought he would work until age fifty-five, then retire to a quiet adult community to play golf. You, on the other hand, never wanted to retire. Your unspoken plan was to keep on working indefinitely and live in a big city with a vibrant cultural life. As you age, your unspoken expectations are about to come into the open, leading to conflict and stress.

Differing expectations concerning wealth and finances. Your wife expected that you would, like her, want to become extremely wealthy and that you would work extremely hard to do so. You, on the other hand, intended to be content with less money and were more interested in spending time at home and investing yourself in the role of parenting and family life.

Good Stress Opportunity #3:
Blame and Anger About the Past

When we bottle up resentment toward our loved ones (about things done or not done, things said or left unsaid) we are creating virtual "land mines" likely to detonate at some point in our future. Here are some common examples:

Resentments about past decisions. Perhaps you resent the fact that your spouse pushed you to move from a house or town you loved. Now you're grieving for the past and deeply angry at your partner.

Blame about "might-have-beens." As you reach your later years and retirement looms, you blame your spouse for not being more of a success. Or you feel that you might have been a successful executive (or musician, or poet, or whatever) if you had not stopped working and stayed home to be the parent who provided most of the care to your children.

Unlocking the Good Stress Within Problems

How can you begin the process of identifying areas of stress in your relationships and, by taking action, make them stronger and more stable?

Take a frank look at areas of stress in your closest relationships. Review your responses from the Personal Stress Inventory. As you review each one (especially those in the Home Life and Routines and Marriage/Love Relationships sections), look for clues to larger issues that you and your significant other could benefit from addressing.

If you have been avoiding a stressful issue, ask why. Have you been afraid of an argument, of losing a friend, of a divorce, or something else? Try to understand the reason the problem has remained unresolved and why it has assumed such weighty dimensions. By balancing that reason against the potential benefits of taking action, you can make a reality-based decision about whether to bring the problem into the open for discussion.

Decide on *underlying* issues to be addressed. Could it be that you are not dealing with one specific stress but with larger issues instead? Are the stresses you identified part of a larger overall pattern? (Perhaps you're not just resentful because your spouse earns more than you; you're deeply angry because your own ambitions have been lost in the relationship.)

Plan appropriate ways to take action to resolve the stress. Should you simply have a conversation with your spouse, friend, or partner? Should you first discuss the problem with a friend or professional counselor before deciding what to do? If you've been living with a problem for some time, there is probably no need to act impulsively now to solve it. Allow yourself the luxury of time to consider different options and make plans.

Taking steps to resolve the stress you've identified requires courage. But as we have discovered, good stress almost always produces positive results when it is resolved. If you truly have discovered a stress that is preventing your relationship from becoming closer and more fulfilling, your courage and efforts will have been very much to the good.

PART III

Minimizing the Damage that Bad Stress Is Causing in Your Life

Before we move to the final section of this book, we need to confront a troubling reality: Not all our bad stresses can be converted to good ones.

Furthermore, not all bad stress can be made to go away according to our personal plans or timetables. Bad stress is often rooted in ongoing life situations that we are powerless to directly control. For example:

▶ You have just been diagnosed with a chronic disease that will require self-monitoring, medical care, and financial hardship.

▶ The company you own is experiencing long-term challenges from foreign competitors.

▶ Your son or daughter just dropped out of college and has a drinking problem that will require professional intervention.

If you weigh such problems against the seven good stress or bad stress laws covered in Chapter 2 of this book, you will see that there really are bad stresses in life.

Yet there is good news regarding bad stresses too. There is a hidden opportunity contained in the concept of fight or flight. Even bad stress can serve as a call to action, a signal that it's time to make things change. Even if a negative stress cannot be eliminated entirely, its pernicious effects can be dramatically reduced through action-taking. Even small actions in the face of chronic bad stress reward us with a sense of relief and personal progress. This is the reason action-taking is the theme that underlies all the strategies suggested in the pages that follow.

When we move ahead in our lives despite bad stresses, we see that they lack the power to destroy us. By taking consistent action, we can still keep our lives stable, satisfying, and profoundly worthwhile.

11

BALANCING YOUR LIFE AROUND BAD STRESSES

When we are confronted with major life problems that cannot be quickly relieved, we have a fundamental choice to make about how we can organize our lives. We can allow our problems to become the centerpiece of our life, coloring and ruining everything around it, or we can surround the problems with many other positive activities and keep our life in a healthy balance.

It sounds like a simple choice. Yet it's worth remembering that when some people are dealing with a chronic source of bad stress, they actually prefer to remain stuck in it and let it throw their lives out of kilter.

The underlying reasons become clearer when we observe how differently people cope with similar chronic stresses.

▶ Patricia, whose husband has advanced Alzheimer's disease, makes daily visits to the care facility where he now lives. She sits by his side for most of the day. Then she goes home, makes dinner for herself, and calls her sister to report about her husband's condition. The next day she repeats the same activities. Arlene, another woman who is in substantially the same situation with a husband who can no longer recognize her or respond, engages in a far wider range of activities. She visits her husband three times a week but is also an avid reader, a member of a bird-watching club, a volunteer at a literacy program for kids, and a member of her church choir. She is dealing responsibly and appropriately with her husband's illness, yet she has kept it from destroying her own life.

❱ A man named Jack has "stuck it out" through many years in a repetitive, uninteresting job with the postal service and is now two years away from retirement. Jack is so angry that on most evenings he drinks more than he should and falls asleep in front of his TV. He is just waiting to retire. Another man named Singh, a college administrator, is in largely the same situation. Singh feels he cannot leave his job because if he does, he will lose a large portion of his pension, but he has taken his life in quite a different direction. He has become self-educated in the area of Italian Renaissance art. He takes courses, travels, and last year even taught a course on the topic at his local adult education center. After retirement he intends to write a book and possibly start a company to lead tours to Italy.

❱ Perry, a man who has diabetes, has concluded that the active part of his life is essentially over because he must now manage a difficult and debilitating disease. He blames himself and says that he brought the disease upon himself by gaining a lot of weight. Yet Sarah, who also has diabetes, had a far different response to her diagnosis. After her initial denial and anger, she started a program of nutrition and regular exercise. She now says she is in the "best shape" of her life and credits diabetes as a wake-up call that told her to get her health back in order.

So we see that there are two basic patterns that can evolve in response to chronic major life stresses. What keeps people from naturally gravitating toward the better, more balanced path? Let's take a closer look.

Guilt

Guilt is one of the major factors that prevents people from rebalancing their lives around chronic problems. Patricia, whose entire life now revolves around her husband's illness, would feel guilty if she allowed herself to enjoy activities that do not directly contribute to her husband's care. She might even fear that if she engages in enjoyable hobbies and pursuits, other people will see her as self-indulgent and frivolous in light of her husband's problems.

Good intentions form the impetus behind such thought patterns. ("I'm giving up everything for my spouse.") Yet upon closer investigation, it becomes clear that this woman is harming herself, and possibly her husband as well, by failing to get her life in healthy balance. She will burn out, become angry, and possibly get sick herself. She may be indulging in self-indulgent (see "Wallowing in the Problem" on page 94) behavior, believing the best way to share her husband's burden is to make herself as miserable as he has become.

The woman who engages in many activities in and around her husband's illness actually stands a better chance of being mentally strong enough to make good decisions and manage his care.

Fear of Change

Some years ago the U.S. Navy found that certain fighter pilots were dying for a very strange reason. When their planes had been hit by enemy fire and were certain to crash, they nonetheless did not eject from their seats. The navy could conclude only that the pilots preferred the familiarity of the cockpit to the uncertainty of the parachute and open air, even though that decision was sure to cause their death.

Of course, that is a rather extreme example of how far people will go to resist change. Yet it does underscore the important message that familiar routines (even very unhealthy ones) often seem less threatening than healthier new ones for the simple reason that they are more familiar.

This explains the different responses that Perry and Sarah had to the news that they had developed diabetes. Perry receded into negativism, preferring to remain inactive and on familiar ground. Sarah, in contrast, realized that she had to cope with her new stress by doing something *differently*. She started to exercise and eat very healthily.

These stories hark back to a principle we have already explored in this book: taking action is the key to dealing with stress in the most healthy way possible. Taking our first steps can be scary, to be sure. But ultimately, dealing with the change is less scary than grappling with a debilitating bad stress with every waking hour.

Wallowing in the Problem

Some people actually seem to relish the major stresses they have to bear in their lives. In some cases, they even let their problems become their personal self-definitions. We see this distinction in Jack and Singh, the two men who are working dull jobs, waiting to retire. Jack has allowed his problem to actually *become* him. Singh balanced his life in and around his dull job and invented entirely new identities for himself as scholar, traveler, and teacher.

The tendency to wallow in a problem also embodies elements of self-blame, especially where midlife health problems such as heart attacks, strokes, and diabetes are concerned. At such times, the sufferer is apt to think, "I did this to myself and now I'm getting what I deserve." There may even be a somewhat macho element to this thinking pattern in which the sufferer thinks that he is "taking his shots" from the problem but will ultimately fight his way out of it if he can stay engaged in the conflict for the long haul.

Wallowing in a problem also has its basis in some good intentions. The struggling individual believes he or she is really dealing with the stress at hand by giving it full attention. Yet as with guilt, the good intentions lead to a less-than-optimal results when life remains out of balance and artificially anchored in bad stress.

Exercise

Take steps to balance your life around a bad stress.

IF you feel the advice in this chapter applies to you because you have allowed a chronic bad stress to take over your life in inappropriate ways, how can you begin to set things straight?

The key is to take action in one small way at a time. "Rebalancing your life," after all, sounds like a complex undertaking. So the key is to start with small, manageable steps and transfer the momentum they bring into affecting more large-scale changes.

Here are some simple steps toward rebalancing that you can probably take today:

Do something you used to love that you have not enjoyed recently. It could be a craft, a bicycle ride, a walk in a favorite spot you haven't visited lately. You'll be reconnecting with a part of yourself, possibly one that deserves reintegration into your life now that you are dealing with a source of ongoing stress.

Engage in a new activity. Visit the new bookstore that just opened in your city or town. Prepare a new recipe for your dinner. Go to your health club and take a tai chi class for the first time. You'll be demonstrating to yourself that you are free to expand your life in new ways.

Change something about your life. Rearrange your bedroom, buy a new stove, or toss out some old clothes and buy some new ones. Even small changes can convince you that you have freedom, even in the face of your problem. You have the ability to adapt to what life brings your way.

Visit or call an old friend. You could say, "I have a problem I want to tell you about" or simply start small by just getting back in touch. Often by talking about all the activities in your life (your kids are in college, your job keeps you busy, you installed new carpets last year) you demonstrate to yourself that the central problem that stresses you really is not the only thing taking place in your life. By talking things through, you might realize that your life is more in balance than you might have believed.

12

IF YOU LEAVE, WILL YOU LEAVE THE BAD STRESS BEHIND?

It's not always possible, but sometimes we can leave a bad boss, quit a bad job, end our negative relationships. However, "walking away" is not always a step to be taken lightly. Are you walking away from a bad situation or failing to confront life issues that need to be resolved? Will you only bring the same problems to the next job, the next town, or the next marriage? Let's take a closer look.

If fight or flight are two options when we are under stress, what's wrong with exercising the second of those two options? In other words, why not escape a bad stress by simply running away?

In some cases, it really *is* possible to resolve negative stresses by eliminating them. Like our earliest ancestors, we can sometimes escape the lion or the bear, or move to higher ground until the forest fire passes.

Yet in our complex lives today, such escape is not usually so simple, as we see in these familiar stories.

▶ After five years in a stressful marriage, a woman summoned up her courage and asked her overbearing husband for a divorce. After the marriage had been dissolved, she blamed her former husband for much of what had gone wrong. Yet she also blamed herself. She wondered whether she had done enough to save her marriage and whether she was really "the marrying kind."

Then, a few years later, she met a man, fell in love, and took the risk of marrying again. This time her marriage worked out beautifully. The frictions that had destabilized her first marriage were simply not present in her second. By getting out of her first marriage, she really had eliminated a major stress and moved to a much better place.

▶ A man had an extremely bad experience in his first job out of college. He felt he was stifled, with no chance to show his abilities. Even worse, he deeply resented his manipulative boss. So he quit and quickly found a new job with a youthful, entrepreneurial firm where he believed he would fit in better. But the change only deepened his problems and stress. After changing jobs, he found himself in a new dead-end job with a new tyrannical boss. Because changing jobs had not let him escape his stresses, he was reluctant to start a new job search and try again.

As we think about these two people, it's tempting to believe that the woman did something right by leaving her first marriage. After all, her new marriage seems to prove there is nothing "wrong" with her. We're also suspicious of the man who can't seem to find the right job. He must have a problem. Maybe he resents authority and has a cocky attitude. Or he's just "green" and needs more real-world experience before he can do well in any job.

Those possibilities are just that. Possibilities. They represent our attempts to define the nature of change. We still need to ask a bigger question: Why is it that sometimes fleeing from problems makes them go away and sometimes flight has no effect.

The Illusion of Control

How can we know when fleeing will bring an end to a bad stress and when it won't?

Part of the answer lies in recognizing the fact that when we make any change in life, we enjoy only partial control over the outcome no matter how much we try to reduce or eliminate the possibility of failure.

> ◗ A boxer who's training for a fight is determined not to repeat the mistakes he made in his last bout. He's looked at the tapes, analyzed what went wrong. He's also spent hours studying the opponent he'll be fighting this time by watching videos of his opponent's previous fights and working with some of his former sparring partners. And, of course, he's in top condition. When he walks into the ring, he'll be ready! Yet who will win? It's anybody's guess. No matter how intelligently this fighter has prepared, he knows all too well that he does not enjoy absolute control over the outcome. His opponent has been making the same preparations he has. Both fighters enjoy only a limited ability to control the outcome.
>
> ◗ A saleswoman is worried because she has not made a sale in the last week. So as she drives to her next sales call, the president of a small company, she goes over everything that's gone wrong in all her sales calls during the last week. She will not make the same mistakes again, she's going to sell this guy! She mentally reviews her presentation, visualizes the sale taking place (a technique she learned in sales training), and walks into the meeting feeling centered and assured. Yet before she can even start her presentation, something surprising happens. The president takes a quick glance at the brochures she's arranged before him and says, "I'm ready to buy." She's made her sale without even trying. Did she even need to prepare?

All our preparations control only one side of any interaction.

In fact, they don't even do that. Our area of control is extremely limited. We believe that when we are doing what we need to do to find a better job, a better marriage, or a better boss, we can actually eliminate the possibility of failure. We believe that with the right kind of preparation, we can avoid the problems that plagued us before.

How much control do we really have? The following chart can help us visualize our ability to control the outcomes as we attempt to escape from stressful situations and move to healthier circumstances.

Our Spheres of Influence

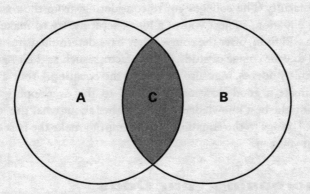

A = the factors we can control as we make changes in our lives

B = the factors we cannot control (controlled by other people, chance, circumstance, etc.)

C = our real sphere of influence

This simple chart tells us something we already know, that life is a process of cooperation, reconciliation, and compromise.

Yet the chart is helpful. It offers a simple way of visualizing the process that really takes place when we attempt to move into new areas we hope will eliminate the causes of our bad stress.

As you take a new job, you try to control everything you can by preparing the skills you'll need, understanding the new company, analyzing what went wrong in your last position, and more. The company, from its side of the equation, tries to control what *it* can by hiring the right person, providing support and training, making the job doable, and more. When your preparation and the company's actions overlap, the area of shared objectives, you have some real control over outcomes.

If you're unhappy with the college you're attending and decide to transfer to another one, you try to control as much as you can as you select a new college to attend. You read the materials, visit the campuses, meet students and members of the faculty. The colleges you're considering, from their side of the equation, subject you to a lot of scrutiny, try to make sure you will fit in, offer the courses they have determined are essential to your course of study. (Other factors, such as their need to recruit students, may also be part of the equation.) Your ability to make a good decision is limited to the overlapping area. Using the best knowledge you can gather about what the "other side" brings to the equation, you attempt to make the best decision you can.

Increasing Your Odds of Making the Right Changes

How can we increase the likelihood that when we move away from bad stress, we will be moving into something better? Using the Spheres of Influence chart on page 101 as a way to help visualize our areas of control, we can arrive at an action plan.

First, we can zero in on factors in the C area. In practical terms, this means identifying a small, well-defined number of issues that really matter the most and negotiating them with the "other side" before committing to making the change.

If you've left a job because you wanted more opportunities

to advance, for example, you can discuss that issue in job interviews with hiring firms. Of if you've determined that you were a victim of discrimination (against women, people of your background or sexual orientation, etc.) in your last job, you can study the new firm carefully to reduce the likelihood that you will encounter the same obstacles again.

You can't control everything the other side brings to the equation (you never can), but with the right focus, you *can* exert control over many critical factors. By doing that, you dramatically increase your odds of success.

Second, we can accept the reality that total control is beyond our reach. This may sound like a frustrating plateau to reach. No matter how diligently we research new situations or study ourselves, we can still be the victims of factors that are beyond our control.

Yet with the right mind-set, this realization can turn out to be *liberating*. That new job, new marriage, new college, or other new circumstance might surprise us in ways we never expected. Often, the B side of the equation contains good elements we did not even know enough to ask about. Perhaps your new wife will not only be kind but will be from a culture that opens up surprising new areas of knowledge and enjoyment in your life. Perhaps your new company will acquire another firm in another state and put you in charge of important new operations. All those surprising "perhaps" elements can make life a lot more interesting.

Sometimes we can move ahead only by realizing that we do not enjoy complete control over what happens to us.

Some people have termed this approach to living *playfulness*.

With a playful outlook, you move ahead and try new things without obsessing about everything we cannot control. Like a football player who advances down the field with the opponent's goalpost squarely in sight, we'd love to run straight ahead toward our goal. Yet we realize we must adjust and adapt along the way, moving around defenders and doing what we need to do as we follow a path that turns out to be anything but straight.

Learning to *progress*, not *obsess*, can be a critical factor in enjoying life more. It makes life not only less tense but more effective too.

Exercise

**Do a "Spheres of Influence" analysis of a
past life change.**

USE the Spheres of Influence diagram on page 101 to analyze two changes you have made in your life, one that
worked out well and one that produced less fortunate outcomes.

Using the chart, map out:

▶ The A factors you could control about the change
   you are making
▶ The B that were controlled by the other people or
   entities involved in making the change
▶ The C factors that represented your real sphere of
   influence

What does this experiment tell you about how effectively
you handled those life changes? Does it offer any insights
on how you might better handle similar life transitions in the
years ahead?

13

BREAKING THE GRIP OF
TYPE A BEHAVIOR

Are you simply stressed, or do you have a type A personality? If you are a true Type A, will your obsessive behavior patterns shorten your life and do you other harm?

Those are troubling questions, but they have surprisingly reassuring answers. Type A behavior doesn't strike unexpectedly in response to stress; it usually appears as a pattern early in life. It is easy to identify and it can often be changed. In this chapter, we'll explore whether Type A patterns have gained control over you. If they have, we'll learn some simple techniques that can help put your life back in balance.

Next to stress itself, Type A behavior may well be the most frequently self-diagnosed psychological ailment in America today. For a relatively academic concept—the term Type A was coined more than twenty-five years ago by two psychologists, Meyer Friedman and Ray H. Rosenman, who also called the syndrome "hurry sickness"—it's remarkable that the theory has come to be so pervasive in people's minds.

Consider these familiar ways we encounter the concept in our daily life:

The obsessive elevator user. A few people are waiting for an elevator in a building lobby. Soon a man cuts to the front, takes over the control panel and pushes the up button once, then twice . . . then five and six times. In unspoken agreement, the same thought is running

through everyone's minds: "This guy is a real Type A."
The horn honker. You're waiting for a stoplight to turn green so you can drive through an intersection, and the moment the light changes, the fellow behind you honks his horn once, then twice, because you are not reacting as quickly as he would like. Again the thought runs through your mind, "Another Type A back there."
The busy signal. One day at work, you dial your home number and find the number busy. Just for the heck of it, you redial the number immediately. (Who knows, maybe your husband or wife was just about to hang up?) It's still busy, so you try again and again. You realize there's no rational reason for behaving this way, but you go on trying anyway. When your partner finally answers, you ask, "Why were you on the phone all that time?" He or she answers, "I was on for only five minutes! What's wrong with you?" You both know the answer to that question—you've had an episode of Type A behavior.

And on and on it goes. We see people behaving in the same compulsive ways in supermarkets, at ATM machines, at our children's sporting events. It seems that Friedman and Rosenman were really onto something. We are a Type A society.

What Is Type A Behavior?

To find the clearest, most concise definition, we need to go back to a 1974 research paper from Friedman and Rosenmann, "The Key Cause—Type A Behavior Pattern."

In their words:

> Type A Behavior Pattern is an action-emotion complex that can be observed in any person who is *aggressively* involved in a *chronic, incessant* struggle to achieve more

> and more in less and less time, and is required to do so,
> against the opposing efforts of other things or other per-
> sons.

That sounds bad—and perhaps it is. Yet in their paper Friedman and Rosenman allay our fears a bit by adding the following statement:

> It is not psychosis or a complex or worries or fears of phobias or obsessions, but a socially acceptable—indeed often praised—form of conflict.

In other words, people become Type A because they are encouraged by our society to do so. Or, at least, Type A people believe they are behaving in socially sanctioned ways.

Why We Obsess About Being Type A

The urge to psychological self-diagnosis is strong within our society. Once we attach the name of a syndrome to the way we behave, we believe we've gained new insights into ourselves. (We can find a book or do some research on the Internet to find out more about ourselves.)

Plus, there is something attractive in the aura that surrounds the idea of being Type A that has attracted the attention of our society:

▶ Type A personalities are high achievers.
▶ Type A personalities are driven—just like our society tells us we should be.
▶ Type A personalities are action-oriented. Unlike all the people who take time to ponder before acting, they know what to do and do it—even if they are acting in compulsive ways.

Yet there is a difference between having a genuine Type A personality and simply being someone who exhibits obsessive behavior patterns from time to time.

Here are some characteristics of Type A patterns that are not well known in our society:

Type A patterns emerge early in life. A hard-driving Type A person who is at the top of his or her company probably began to exhibit the behavior long before—perhaps in school or an early job. The Type A person won rewards for driving hard and unrelentingly—or at least so he or she believes. Because the behavior was encouraged, it has become second nature.

The behavior usually flares up in response to a specific outside stimulus. The behavior materializes when something happens to trigger it. It might be a lost object around the house that becomes the object of a frenzied four-hour search—or a slow-moving line at the bank or phone messages that are not returned.

In short, any object or situation that fails to yield quickly can become the epicenter of the obsessive attention. Considered this way, we see that Type A behavior is akin to stress addiction. When something does not yield, obsessive, stressful reactions escalate.

Needless to say, unchecked patterns of Type A behavior can be very hard on the people who are in the vicinity of the Type A person—family, friends, colleagues, staff, and so on. Yet the Type A person rarely perceives all the havoc he or she is exerting on others. In the Type A person's eyes, he or she is behaving in a positive and highly effective way, perhaps better than everyone else. Success has been built upon acting just this way. Because the behavior is so ingrained, it is often invisible to its victim.

What About Type B Behavior?

With all the attention Type A behavior attracts, it is easy to forget that the researchers who first identified it also identified a corresponding behavior pattern: Type B behavior. To quote again from their original paper:

> **The person with Type B Behavior Pattern is the exact opposite of the Type A subject. He, unlike the Type A person, is rarely harried by desires to obtain a wildly increasing number of things or participate in an endlessly growing series of events in an ever decreasing amount of time. His intelligence may be as good as or even better than that of the Type A.** *Similarly,* **his ambition may be as great or even greater than that of his Type A counterpart . . . He may also have a considerable amount of "drive," but its character is such that it seems to steady him, give confidence and security to him, rather than to goad, irritate, and infuriate, as with the Type A man.**

Would You Rather Be Type A or Type B?

This question is, of course, somewhat misleading because we have more than two choices in life: to be either Type A or Type B. But the existence of the two types represents a call to find balance and equilibrium in our lives—and to live as masters of our life's pacing rather than its slaves.

If you believe you may have fallen victim to Type A patterns (and remember, such patterns are often difficult for the sufferer to observe), you might be well advised to engage in some self-scrutiny and self-examination, for some very good reasons. First, a Type A life is one that is often led at the beck and call of stress.

Some Type A sufferers are stressed all the time—the true victims of Friedman and Rosenman's "hurry sickness." For others, the behavior is triggered only in response to some external obstacle: when a client will not return calls, the electrician fails to arrive on time, or when the child will not quickly finish up his homework. At such times, Type A patterns emerge and we are suddenly miserable, humbled by stress, and those around us suffer. Chronic Type A sufferers experience an especially intense level of stress that may make them especially vulnerable to high blood pressure, stroke, and all the other physical ailments associated with stress.

Are You Type A? How to Uncover Type A Behavior in Yourself

Here are a few self-diagnostic techniques that can help determine if you have fallen victim to Type A behavior:

Keep a log of your daily activities for a few days—perhaps as long as one week. Divide a sheet of paper into fifteen-minute time blocks. Keep a watch or clock visible and, at the end of each brief period, jot a note about what you did. A large number of compulsive, repeated tasks may indicate that you switch into Type A behavior in response to obstacles.

A time log can reveal some even more conclusive signs of Type A patterns, such as your inability to meet your two or three biggest priorities on any given day, because you are acting reactively, in response to obstacles as they arise.

Monitor your reactions to life's obstacles and setbacks. Sadly, there are no shortage of them in our daily lives. We're often stuck in traffic, put on hold, left waiting for luncheon partners who are themselves stuck in traffic and arrive late— and on and on the list goes. Try to observe yourself at such times. Do you obsessively latch on to the problem and try to break your way through it even when you know it is beyond your control? Or do you, like a Type B, turn your attention to other things for a while before returning to the obstacle?

Freeing Yourself from Compulsive Patterns

By its very definition, Type A behavior is deeply ingrained. The person suffering from it may even believe that he or she has been rewarded for it. For such reasons, Type A patterns can be hard to chase away.

The key is to consciously try to emulate Type B behavior when obstacles intrude. The unanswered doorbell, the long line at the gas pumps—with a little awareness, you can see these as opportunities to behave in noncompulsive ways.

Actively practice self-disruptive behavior. Instead of butting your head time and time again against the "triggering" obstruction that lies in your path, consciously turn your attention to something else. Take out a file of papers you are working on and focus on that. Or look at the clock and decide you will wait five minutes before trying to make that phone call again. In time, Type A patterns can be reeducated away as you experience a welcome sense of relief that accompanies the release of negative stressors in your lire.

Try organizing your way in a Type B pattern. Set aside large time blocks when you will tackle your one or two most important projects each day. It might mean working a morning at home each week so you can complete a big written report, or setting aside a day to complete a household project instead of weaving it in and around a weekend's many commitments. As you organize yourself in this different, nonhabitual way, pay attention to the rewards you are gaining. The quality of your work may improve, or you may bring a higher level of creativity to your activity.

Fight the tendency to judge yourself on your numbers. This is another aspect of Type A behavior—the tendency to judge personal accomplishments on numbers alone. How many calls did you return? Did you close $1 million in sales last month? Did you sew more costumes than anyone else for your daughter's ballet-class performance of *The Nutcracker*? Remind yourself that there are other ways to judge what you do. Perhaps you did not close five sales last week but you did improve relations with several important clients and showed them your new product line. Perhaps you did not complete the most costumes for your daughter's show, but you spent some meaningful time with her as you worked together. As you try to stretch yourself in these new, qualitative directions, you may find that greater satisfactions lie in Type B patterns than you expected.

Set aside concerns of rankings and status. Type A people believe—consciously or unconsciously—that they are at the top of the heap because they act the way they do. They must be best because they did the most. Strive to remind yourself that excellence may not reside in the numbers. You might be the best husband because of the quality of communication with your wife, not because you make the most money. You might be the best executive because you are an inspiring leader to your staff, not because you generate the most dollars.

14

RECOVERING FROM TRAUMATIC STRESS

We all would like to make ourselves immune to life's major catastrophes. Yet no life is free of all misfortunes. When they strike, they can deal us blows from which we recover only after a great deal of time and pain.

As unpleasant as it is, let's consider how we can deal effectively with traumatic, stressful events such as these:

- The death of a loved one
- The onset of a serious chronic disease afflicting ourselves or a loved one
- A divorce or the end of an important relationship
- The sudden loss of a job after many years
- A miscarriage
- An operation, handicap, or illness that alters our level of activity in the world

Such stresses have the ability to unsettle and disturb us. Who among us has not had a car accident, a fire or robbery in the home, a child flunk out of college, or a sudden financial setback?

Applying the DABDA Model

When dealing with such extreme stresses, many people have found helpful advice in the writings of Dr. Elisabeth Kubler-Ross, especially her book *On Death and Dying*. It was Dr. Kubler-Ross who developed the DABDA model (standing for

Denial and Isolation, Anger, Bargaining, Depression, and Acceptance) to explain the predictable stages we can expect to go through when recovering from a significant life loss or change.

In such circumstances, Dr. Kubler-Ross states, we tend to go through five predictable DABDA stages:

▶ **Denial and Isolation.** We have a sudden ostrichlike reaction when faced with life-altering news that doesn't fit into our sense of who we are. We try to stick our heads in the sand and say, "This has not happened! This can't be happening to me! This is not who I am!"

  Most people who have been through stressful events are familiar with this pattern. The day after the death of a loved one, for example, we tell ourselves "This didn't happen! My loved one is going to walk through the door any moment and that will be the end of all this nonsense!" Or after we learn we have a serious disease, we think, "They mixed up the lab results! The phone is going to ring and it will all be straightened out!" After time, however, such denial is difficult to maintain and we soon move on to the next DABDA plateau.

▶ **Anger.** In this stage we get furious. We fire questions at ourselves, at everyone who will listen, and many people who will not: "Why me? This is unfair! What did I do to deserve this problem? Why is my life getting completely torn apart in this way?" If we are religious, we might get angry at God. (After all, God is supposed to protect us from harm.) Or we blame our spouses, children, friends, or family members for our new problems.

▶ **Bargaining.** In this stage we think thoughts such as "Maybe I can put my marriage back together! This has been a bad interlude, but maybe we can talk. Okay, is that a deal?" Or we think, "Okay, the stress test showed that I have a coronary blockage, but I don't need an angioplasty! I can reverse it and be good as new if I watch my diet. Isn't that so?"

Some bargaining is effective, some less so. Yet in either case it serves as a needed step in the healing process, moving us into a rational, problem-solving mode. We are testing reality and starting to grapple with the issues surrounding how we will change and restructure our lives in the wake of the stressful event. Yet more adjustments follow.

▶ **Depression.** In this stage we get very "down" as we admit the possibility that our life really will not get back to the way it was before the stressful event occurred. Many people lose hope, experience trouble sleeping, or see a drop in energy or sex drive. Still others lose any sense of the future. It is just impossible to imagine life going on after such a traumatic change. ("I will never be successful after losing my job" or "My spouse was the love of my life, which is now over.")

But after we have gone to this dark place and dwelled there for a while, the gloom begins to lift and we can move on to the next phase.

▶ **Acceptance.** We reluctantly admit the possibility that our lives will now go on in a new, altered fashion. We can even see new possibilities and options. Life will never be the same, but it just might be a life worth living after all.

Why DABDA Helps Us

Not everyone experiences the DABDA steps sequentially as outlined above. The model simply provides a diagram for what we are experiencing in response to cataclysmic life changes. At the same time, it can be comforting to know that other people have already been through a process similar to the one we are passing through.

Knowing about DABDA also lessens the likelihood that we will become stalled at one stage of the recovery process and not move on. It's seductive, for instance, to go on living in the false security of denial. Or to dwell in our anger, casting ourselves as victims of an unfair and vindictive world. Yet if we are able to realize where we stand in the DABDA process of recovery, we stand a much better chance of moving on out of stress and finding new satisfaction in life.

It is also helpful to know that people usually bounce back and forth around the DABDA stages, because the process does not always move in a sequential, orderly way. One day you may be working on issues of acceptance, then become wildly angry the next. Or you might be bargaining on Monday, then experiencing acute depression by midweek.

Recovering from traumatic stress can never be easy. But with the right knowledge and mental outlook, you can move from stress onward to an altered life that is both workable and meaningful. The bad stresses, even the worst of them, will not be powerful enough to permanently throw your life out of balance.

Exercise

Do a DABDA analysis of a past traumatic event in your life.

RECALL a traumatic event from your past and consider how the DABDA steps were played out as you put your life back together.

Chances are that this exercise will uncover some of your personal patterns and predilections for processing stress. If you entered a prolonged period of denial (or depression, or anger) after a past traumatic event, you might tend to do the same thing in response to difficult events in the future. Knowing such personal tendencies might help you adapt to future life calamities with less pain.

15

CLASSIC TOOLS
FOR STRESS REDUCTION

If you visit a bookstore or library, you'll find many books that deal exclusively with the stress-reduction techniques in this chapter. There are books on meditation, exercise, herbal remedies, inner peace, biofeedback, and much, much more.

Since no book on stress would be complete without information on these techniques, we present them for you here. Please bear in mind that not all the techniques will work for you, but one or two of them might help you reduce the sensations of the chronic bad stress that you are living with at this point in your life. Explore those that appeal to you. Good luck!

Practice Meditation

Meditation is a simple and pleasant mind-quieting technique with origins in Hindu religious practice. One form of meditation, Transcendental Meditation, was widely popularized back in the 1960s when a guru named Maharishi Mahesh Yogi established TM centers in cities and on campuses across the United States, Canada, and Europe. The one way to learn TM as taught by the maharishi was to take instruction at one of these centers, some of which are still in operation today.

Then in 1975 *The Relaxation Response,* a best-selling book by psychologist named Dr. Herbert Benson, taught millions of Americans how to practice a similar system of meditation without the need to visit a center or take formal instruction. In the years since, meditation has entered the mainstream of American thinking. It has even become possible to take a class at your local adult school or Y, if you so desire.

Meditation has retained its popularity for some very good reasons. Many of the people who like the technique report the following benefits:

- Since meditation is usually practiced upon arising, they start their days with a calmer attitude and less nervousness
- A better ability to cope calmly with life's daily stresses
- Better sleeping patterns
- More relaxed and satisfying sexual relationships
- In some cases, an improvement in stress-related physical problems such as high blood pressure, stomach upsets, and other digestive ailments

One of the best things about meditation is that you can simply try it and see if it works for you. Following are two types of meditation.

Mantra-Based Meditation

Select a word (a "mantra") that you will repeat silently to yourself as you meditate. It could be a pleasant-sounding one- or two-syllable word that has no meaning to you (examples: uma, aba, ila.) In his book *The Relaxation Response,* Dr. Benson suggests simply using the word "one."

Find a place where you will not be interrupted while you meditate. Your bedroom, a study, even the train you take to and from work, can serve you as good meditating locales.

Sit in a comfortable position in bed, in a chair, or on the floor if that is comfortable for you. Put your hands in your lap. Close your eyes.

Begin to repeat your mantra to yourself. The overall experience should be easy and pleasant. Silently repeat your word and, if your mind drifts away from it, gently start again without thinking that you "did something wrong." The mantra functions in a fascinating way by temporarily giving our mind's thought- and word-generating processes something to "chew on." Instead of thinking about problems, we are humming along on our mantra. It's a feeling that can be very pleasant. Many people who meditate report that as soon as a few days after beginning meditation, starting to meditate by using their mantras leads them into a deeply relaxing or even trancelike state.

Meditate for about twenty minutes. Don't use an alarm, just place a wristwatch in your hand where you can refer to it, or sit where you can watch a clock. When you are done with your mantra-based meditation, allow yourself a few relaxing minutes before you get up and start other activities.

Try to meditate twice a day. The ideal, according to practitioners, is to meditate once just after you awake in the morning and once before dinner at night. Many meditators do not like to meditate after eating, but it is a highly individual thing.

Breathing-Based Meditation

Follow the instructions for mantra-based meditation but instead of concentrating on a word as you meditate, concentrate on your breathing. People who like breathing-based meditation offer the following pointers on the technique:

As you sit in a comfortable position, try placing a hand flat on your stomach, just below your navel. Breathe calmly and comfortably "into" this hand as you meditate.

Experiment with different breathing "counts." You might try breathing in to a slow count of three, then out again to the same count; or in to a count of three and then out to a count of two. Concentrating on these patterns is said to exert a calming effect on the mind and body. Like the nonsense syllable used in the mantra-based meditation described above, it can lead your mind away from thoughts about daily issues and lead to a state of deep relaxation.

To learn more about meditation:

- ➤ Visit the Transcendental Meditation Web site at *www.tm.org* or call 1-888-LEARNTM in the continental United States to find a TM center in your area.
- ➤ Read *The Relaxation Response* by Dr. Herbert Benson

Try Biofeedback

Biofeedback uses a device (usually electronic, but not always) to monitor what is going on with your body and your brain. An advanced biofeedback device might give you continual readings on your heart rate, blood pressure, body temperature, galvanic skin response, sweating, temperature, and even your brain waves. A simpler device might monitor only one or two of these activities. The idea behind biofeedback is to monitor these indicators as you practice deep breathing or relaxing thoughts, seeking thinking techniques that help to reduce stress. Sometimes biofeedback users report that simply monitoring what's taking place in their bodies while relaxing produces feelings of relaxation and lowered stress.

Biofeedback can be practiced in the office of a biofeedback practitioner. It is now becoming more possible to practice it at home, thanks to a number of small, inexpensive self-monitoring devices that have recently become available such as the GSR2, a galvanic skin response-monitoring device that retails for about $80.

Bear in mind, too, that there are no-cost ways to experiment with biofeedback by using devices you might already have in your home. You can simply use your watch to count your number of heartbeats per minute. While continuing to monitor for five minutes, try some deep breathing or relaxing thoughts (such as meditating on a mantra or imagining yourself in a pleasant locale) to see whether you can find a way to use your thinking to lower your pulse rate. If you own a device to measure your blood pressure, you can use it before a five-minute meditation period (or a period of deep breathing) and then afterward to see whether your mental activities have lowered your pressure, a sign of lowered stress.

Biofeedback isn't for everyone. But if it works for you, it might serve as a useful tool in your stress-monitoring and stress-fighting arsenal.

To learn more about biofeedback:

➤ Visit Biofeedbackzone, an Internet retailer that sells bio-feedback books, training materials and supplies, at *www. biofeedbackzone.com*.

Be Sure to Get Enough Sleep

Lack of sleep or troubled sleep can be a major contributor to our ability to cope with all the stresses in our lives. How much sleep is enough? The National Sleep Foundation states that in general, most adults need an average of seven to nine hours of sleep a night. Some of us can't perform at our peak unless we've slept a full ten hours.

How can you determine if you're not sleeping enough? According to the NSF, you're not getting enough sleep if you:

- Have difficulty staying awake or alert during meetings or monotonous situations
- Experience irritability with co-workers, family or friends
- Have difficulty concentrating or remembering facts
- Experience drowsiness when driving or riding in a car

If those indicators show you could use more sleep, here are some steps to follow, adapted from NSF guidelines:

▶ Increase your sleep time gradually over a few weeks. Don't expect to suddenly add several hours. Instead, retire a bit earlier than usual and try to rise a bit later if your schedule permits.

▶ Maintain your new sleep schedule even on weekends.

▶ Avoid caffeine and alcohol in the late afternoon and evening.

▶ Exercise will help you rest better and longer, but schedule your workout at least three hours before bedtime to avoid feeling energized.

▶ Don't nap during the day even if you feel tired. It only makes it harder to fall asleep at night.

▶ If you have trouble falling asleep because you've gone to bed earlier than usual, don't stay in bed and toss and turn. Get up and enjoy a relaxing activity such as listening to music or reading until you feel sleepy, then go to bed again.

To learn more about sleep:

➤ Visit the National Sleep Foundation's Web page at *www.sleepfoundation.org*.

➤ Read *The Promise of Sleep: A Pioneer in Sleep Medicine Explores the Vital Connection Between Health, Happiness, and a Good Night's Sleep* by William C. Dement and Christopher Vaughan.

Exercise

In addition to its many other health benefits, exercise helps us reduce anxiety and depression, sleep better, and have a keener mental outlook. If you are not already exercising, try these suggestions to help you get started with a program of exercise you will enjoy and stay with:

▶ Find a kind of exercise you can reasonably add to your schedule. Decide whether early mornings, lunch hours, or after-work hours really fit best in your schedule. If you're so busy that none of these suggestions works for you, pay special attention to the next suggestion.

▶ Blend exercise in and around your regular daily activities. If your office is on the third or fourth floor, skip the elevator and walk up at least twice a day. If you park your car in the company lot, choose a parking spot well away from the building's entrance. If you commute home by train, get off one station before yours and walk the extra distance two or three times a week. Another good approach is to "multitask" exercise while doing something that is already part of your schedule. Ride an exercise bicycle while you are watching television, for example, or do some stretching while waiting for your e-mail to download. By multitasking in this way, you can include exercise in your daily routine without needing to find extra time.

▶ Consider working with a training partner. When a friend is waiting for you to share a morning run or trip to the exercise room, you have a higher level of motivation to keep going. Having a friend there also makes workouts more pleasant.

▶ Don't approach exercising in a stressful way. If you're jogging one morning and it feels exhausting and difficult instead of fun and stimulating, knock off early and try again in a few days. If you've decided to swim three mornings a week and you miss a day, don't feel that you have "failed" and might as well quit.

Committed exercisers confirm that a healthy dose of self-forgiveness is one of the keys to maintaining an exercise program for the long term.

Avoid Excessive Alcohol and Caffeine

No one has proven that moderate enjoyment of alcohol or coffee contributes to ill health or stress. The key word, obviously, is *moderate*. If you sleep too little and need three cups of strong coffee to get you moving in the morning, that is obviously not a healthy pattern to develop. Or if you need three stiff drinks to calm down each evening upon arriving home from your job, you are using alcohol as a drug to counter the ill effects of stress. Again, that is not a healthy pattern to adhere to.

If you are overusing caffeine or alcohol to control your energy and moods, here are some steps to ease into healthier habits:

For caffeine . . .

Cut back gradually. Going "cold turkey" can lead to headaches, digestive problems such as diarrhea or constipation, and disrupted sleeping patterns. Many people report that they have painlessly reduced their coffee intake by starting the day with their usual cup, then shifted to noncaffeinated tea, decaffeinated coffee, or another beverage.

Try to replace coffee with another beverage you enjoy. Many of the joys of coffee-drinking lie in the rituals and routines that surround it: stopping by a favorite coffee shop on the way to your office, enjoying a cup as you check your morning e-mails, etc. Allowing another beverage to take the place of coffee in those same routines can make the process of caffeine reduction far easier.

Seek professional help if needed. Rather than slipping back and starting to drink heavy coffee again when you encounter withdrawal-related problems, address the problems with a call or visit to your physician. You don't have to go it alone.

For alcohol . . .

As with coffee, make your life change toward lighter drinking gradual. Instead of substituting mineral water for your first beer or glass of wine upon arriving home, go ahead and enjoy your accustomed first drink. But then shift to a nonalcoholic beverage.

Notice and appreciate the benefits of drinking less. Upon arising each morning, remind yourself that you feel clearer and more energetic now that you are limiting your use of alcohol.

Couple your alcohol-reducing program with some healthy activities such as exercising or dieting. When lowering alcohol intake is only one of several life-improving incentives you're engaged in, your chances of success are greater.

Be ready to own up to deeper patterns of alcohol dependency. Alcohol, it is well known, is a strong drug. It is so strong that when people become dependent, they often deny that fact to themselves and those around them. This advice is intended for people who are not alcoholics but who have simply fallen into the habit of having a few more drinks than is healthy. If you feel you are not in that category, that you have developed a real drinking problem, you owe it not only to your stress-reduction program but to your life as a whole to speak with your physician and seek competent assistance in recovery.

To learn more about relying less on caffeine and alcohol:

➤ Read *Caffeine Blues: Wake Up to the Hidden Dangers of America's #1 Drug* by Stephen Cherniske; *Buzz: The Science and Lore of Alcohol and Caffeine* by Stephen Braun, or one of the many books about reducing consumption of alcohol and caffeine.

Try Massage or Acupuncture

A professional massage can be an excellent way to reduce tension and stress. There are so many varieties of massage—shiatsu, Swedish massage and acupressure, to name just a few—it is beyond the scope of this book to describe them all. Another option that's not for everyone is acupuncture, the Chinese medical discipline in which thin needles are inserted into various nerve points in the body to reduce feelings of tension and stress. (Acupuncture has even been shown to be effective in reduction of high blood pressure, cholesterol, and other medical conditions.)

If you are interested in trying massage therapy or acupuncture for stress reduction, consult your local Yellow Pages to see what options are available in your area.

To learn more about massage, acupuncture and similar techniques:

➤ Visit the American Massage Therapy Association's Web page at *www.amtamassage.org*. This site provides referrals to massage therapists in all areas of North America and abroad.

➤ Visit the American Academy of Medical Acupuncture's Web page at www.medicalacupuncture.org.

➤ Read one of the many books on all varieties of massage.

Take Herbs to Reduce Feelings of Stress

A survey done by *Prevention* magazine in 1997 found that one-third of all adult Americans, roughly 60 million people in all, frequently use herbal remedies. The survey also found that each adult American spends an average of $54 on herbs each year. That's a national expenditure of about $3.2 billion.

Many people have expressed interest in a variety of herbs to reduce feelings of stress and anxiety. A partial list includes:

- Ginseng—respected for its abilities to boost energy and immunity, ginseng is also used by many to increase mental and physical stamina in times of difficulty or stress.
- Licorice—widely used in ancient times as a medication, licorice remains one of the most widely dispensed medications in China. Said to treat respiratory problems as well as reduce stress.
- Poria cocos (fu ling)—another traditional Chinese herb used to fight insomnia and nervousness.
- St. John's wort—this herb, used as an antidepressant and stress reducer, has gained widespread notoriety in the American media.
- Vitamin C—vitamin C is not believed to be a stress fighter per se. However, studies have shown that stress and hard physical activity cause Vitamin C to be eliminated quickly from the body. For this reason, it may be a good idea to maintain an intake of Vitamin C (from citrus fruit or in tablet form) during stressful periods in order to uphold your body's defenses against disease.

Remember that it is always prudent to speak with your physician before starting to take these or any other herbs. Although "natural," they are drugs nonetheless and may impact negatively on certain conditions or cause harmful interactions with other medications. There is also the problem of manufacture and regulation: The quality and quantity of specific herbs found in herbal remedies found at health-food stores, pharmacies, etc., has been found to vary considerably.

To learn more about herbal stress remedies:

> ➤ Do some searching on the Internet, while being aware that companies that distribute herbal preparations are apt to make exaggerated claims for the effectiveness of the remedies that they sell. One impartial and very useful Web page is *www.familydoctor.org*, which offers a searchable database of different herbs, their uses, and possible dangers. Another useful Web page is *www.healthfinder.gov*, a government-sponsored source of information on drugs and drug interaction.
>
> There are many books on herbs available at bookstores and libraries. Some are excellent, others offer exaggerated claims for certain herbal preparations. One of the better impartial guides is *The New Encyclopedia of Herbs and Their Uses* by Deni Brown. But with a little searching, you will find other good guides as well.

Live Simply

In the last few years, a number of books have appeared about simplicity. There is also a magazine, *Real Simple,* dedicated to the topic of living in an uncomplicated way. Believers in simplicity tell us that when they make their lives less complicated, they experience less stress and more fulfillment. There is good reasoning behind such claims. When our lives are uncomplicated, there are fewer things to distract us from the activities that bring us the most enjoyment.

Some of the central beliefs of the simplicity movement are:

- ❯ Try to streamline your life routines by cutting down on activities that don't bring you pleasure or serve a useful purpose.
- ❯ Eliminate clutter in your home.
- ❯ Try to find simpler approaches to daily activities such

as cooking, errands, cleaning, gardening, etc.
▶ Reduce the number of possessions you own to the essentials.

To learn more about simplicity:

➤ Read *Simplify Your Life: 100 Ways to Slow Down and Enjoy the Things That Really Matter* by Elaine St. James.

16

DON'T LET WORRY
MAKE BAD STRESS WORSE

Most of the stresses we discussed in this book come from the outside: the bad bosses, ringing phones, traffic jams. What about stresses that come from the inside, the anxieties we create for ourselves?

Of all self-imposed stresses, worry is by far the most pervasive. Worry is a stress in its own right. Yet it also functions on a second and more damaging level by magnifying all the other stresses in our lives, making them appear bigger and bigger until they loom as insurmountable obstacles.

- On the job you have to confront a worker about how much time he spends on the phone making personal calls. You delay the conversation, you worry about it, and soon you're stewing about it all the time.
- You have an appointment next week with a professor to discuss how you can get a low grade improved. Your mind begins to play and replay different scenarios about how the conversation might go. Soon you start to lose sleep over it.
- You made a bad decision a year ago and started a business with a partner whom you didn't know well enough. Relations are now strained and you realize that you are obsessing about the problem on weekends, evenings, and even while you are cooking dinner or going shopping with your kids.

In these common situations, we witness worry's unique power to take something bad and make it a lot worse. Yet the good news is, most worry is founded more on upon illusions than upon reality. When we act on the problem that is causing us to think obsessively, the illusions often disappear, taking worry with them.

Reduce "What-If" Thinking

At one time or another, most of us have been the victim of obsessive thought patterns that lead us down ever-darkening hallways into a virtual labyrinth of obsessive worry.

If you are about to ask your boss for a raise, *what if* he grills you over budget issues? If he does that, *what if* he attacks you about your failure to rein in your staff's travel expenditures in the first quarter of last year? *What if* he then demands that you fire two members of your staff who cost you the most in travel dollars.

What if . . . what if . . . what if.

One "what-if" consideration leads quickly to another and it can be impossible to break free. You're caught in a chain of scenarios for events that will probably never happen.

The lure of the "what-if" pattern is the unspoken belief that through worrying, you will be able to control the outcome of what is about to happen to you. You think you are planning when you start to play out all those scenarios, but in reality you are obsessing. Even when we realize this is the case, we are often unable to break free of the pattern's hold.

One very effective approach is to create a "worst-case" scenario by asking "what's the worst thing that can happen?" This technique is effective because it turns "what-if" thinking back upon itself. Simply dwell on one of the terrible outcomes you are dreading. If your boss confronts you on budget issues, what's the worst thing that can happen? You might have the opportunity to document your department's current expenditures and show that you now have the problem under control. Very specifically, what's the worst thing that could happen if you tell your partner that your agreement isn't working out and you need to part ways? Would you lose the $3,000 you invested? Would you have the chance to buy her out and own a business you now control?

By making your worries reality-based in this way, you break the obsessive patterns and can often begin to take the next step.

Stop Obsessing, Start Planning

Obsessive worrying is really false planning. When we fall victim to its lure, we set up a series of false scenarios and fantasize about how we will behave when they occur. In effect, we are doing little more than creating a series of paper tigers, one after the other, to cower before.

There is a way to harness all the mental energy of worrying and put it to good use, and that is to *plan*. What is the difference between worrying and planning? Simply that planning is more focused and more reality-based. When we worry, we conjure up a storm cloud of undifferentiated, nonspecific problems. When we plan, we select just a few well-defined, specific problems and plan for them strategically. Best of all, the shift from worry to planning is often quite easy to make, a simple matter of directing your mind toward likely problems you might face instead of letting it wander over imaginary ones.

When you find yourself obsessing over a problem, you can take steps like these:

❭ If you're worrying about having a conversation with a loan officer about refinancing your house because you've made some late credit-card payments over the last few years, make a plan. You could first call the bank to ask which credit reports they use in evaluating applications; then obtain a copy of those reports and review them yourself; then contact any credit-card companies who have filed negative information about you to ask how you can get those figures improved *before* you apply to refinance your home. You could even call the bank's loan officer before your meeting to ask what kind of documentation the bank will require to approve a loan in spite of some late credit-card payments on credit reports.

▶ If you've learned that a real estate developer has obtained a tract of land in your town and plans to build a condominium complex that will erode the value of homes in your neighborhood, you can shift that anxiety and worry to positive action, as people in such circumstances often do: You can meet with town officials to find out the procedures the developer must go through before getting approval to build; investigate how similar condominium developments have affected property values in other towns; and further define the problems you are facing. You might also make some calls to locate some lawyers who have represented property owners in similar cases. Now that your problem is better defined and you have obtained expert help, you might organize a neighborhood committee and combat the development in a structured way.

Throwing Caution to the Wind

After some careful planning, you will find that you experience a new sensation of preparedness, calm, and efficacy. The problems that were causing you to obsess only a short time ago now seem to be within your power because you have defined and addressed them.

You might even find that you are now quite comfortable entering into the difficult, stressful situations you were dreading. You know the problems that are likely to arise, and you know how you will deal with them when they do. You are like a sailor who has armed him or herself with good knowledge and good equipment. Is it possible that you can set out for a quiet sail and suddenly find yourself dealing with a storm that blows up unexpectedly? Of course it is. But you need not worry about that too much, because you know you have the skills and knowledge to make on-the-spot decisions that will let you come through unscathed.

Special Problem: Fear of the Unknown

At this point I'd like to explore an especially troubling stress: fear about the outcomes of future events we cannot control. Much as we would like to insulate ourselves from this kind of stress, life often seems to have other plans for us that cause us to stress and worry obsessively for very realistic reasons.

- You're meeting with your physician next Tuesday to learn the results of extensive medical tests that might tell you that you have cancer. You can't do anything but wait day by day. Your uncertainty and anxiety grow to the breaking point.
- Next week your husband, who is in the military, will get on a troop transporter and go overseas to be stationed in a conflict-ravaged foreign country. You are petrified and cannot stop worrying about what could happen to him during his tour of duty there.

Even when such stresses resolve in a positive way (you learn you do not have cancer; your husband returns home safe), they are still not *good* stresses. The severity of possible outcomes is extreme and you cannot stop worrying. It would be irrational to believe that you *could*.

What is the best means of handling such extreme stresses

well? Interestingly, some of our most basic human capabilities can be the most effective of all.

Rely on friends and loved ones to support you instead of toughing it out alone. If you can admit your vulnerability, you actually make yourself stronger and better equipped to confront the challenges ahead.

Seek out a community of support. If your spouse is about to go overseas on a tour of military duty, find a way to connect with other spouses who are facing the same situation you are. Or if you learn you really do have cancer, ask at once to be made part of a support network of other patients. Community, one of the most basic human needs, has a remarkable power to see us through life's most difficult times.

Rely on sources of spiritual support. Times of adversity are those when you might do well to call upon your religion or religious leaders. Prayer or meditation can also help to pull you through the stressful time you are encountering.

Connect with art, nature, and sources of personal inspiration. A trip to a museum or a walk outdoors might go a long way toward reassuring you that things will turn out well. During one of the most difficult times of my own life, after my parents had died and I was emptying their house and dreading the prospect of selling it, I listened almost every day to the Brahms Piano Concerto No. 1. It seemed to express embody all the emotions I was feeling at the time. It was deeply reassuring and it really pulled me through. I'd encourage you to seek out your own sources of reassurance like that when hard times hit.

Keep on hoping. Hope, which appears insignificant in the face of great adversity, is probably a lot stronger than we realize. It's interesting to note that people who have survived foreign prisons, shipwrecks, plane crashes, civil unrest, and other calamities almost always say the same thing afterward: "I never gave up hope." There is apparently much power in those simple words.

Perform a "post mortem" on a problem you were once worrying about.

RECALL a situation that really had you crippled with worry. Perhaps . . .

- you were facing an interview at the college that was your number one choice and you had no idea what questions you would be asked
- you had to fire someone at work
- you had to speak with a neighbor about an addition she had put on her home that was in violation of town code

Think about that situation for a few minutes, then create a quick balance sheet about your worries at the time. On one side of a piece of paper, write down all the things you were obsessing about before the situation occurred. (You were consumed with the idea that the person you were about to fire would become violent, or convinced that the college interviewer would ask you about the French Revolution or the Renaissance.) On the other side of the page, write down what actually happened. In this way, you will see that worrying almost always creates false fears and exaggerated expectations.

This is a liberating exercise that reveals worry for what it is: a fear-based, obsessive pattern that causes us to lose sight of the fact that we are well equipped to overcome many of the obstacles that life places before us.

17

REDUCING
DAILY STRESSES AT WORK

Our jobs present us with many good stresses in disguise. Where else can tension help us accomplish important things, expand our abilities, lead groups of people, earn a livelihood, and more? Yet along with the good, most all jobs also bring negative stresses such as these that we have to accept:

▶ Constant interruptions
▶ A chronic rush to accomplish our most important priorities on any given day
▶ Duties that are especially unpleasant
▶ Difficult relationships with bosses, colleagues and the people we supervise
▶ "Work/life conflict" between our jobs and our personal lives

Let's take a look at some solutions that can serve as immediate stress-fighters in each of these areas.

If You Are Constantly Interrupted

Interruptions are a major stress in most of our workdays. They keep us from tackling our most important jobs and, even worse, make us feel distressed and out of control because our time is not our own, but everyone else's.

These techniques can reduce the stress of interruptions and significantly break their hold on our time:

❱ Adopt focused interruption-preventing techniques. If people report to you, ask them to wait until they have three or more questions "bunched up" before knocking on your door. Also "manage by walking around," visiting people where they work and answering their questions *before* they interrupt you with them. As you walk around, be a keen observer. If a staff member has piles of unanswered phone-message slips on his desk or if he hasn't read a week's backlog of memos in his inbox, you have discovered a problem. By helping that staff member at once, you efficiently tackle problems while they are still small and reduce future interruptions.

❱ Delegate not just work but authority. When you tell people that they have the leeway to make more decisions without consulting you, you prevent interruptions before they occur. The truth is, the more you "micromanage" and hover over every detail of your staff's workload, the more stress *you* accumulate.

❱ Hold regular meetings where staff members can bring up work-related concerns without knocking on your door.

It can be difficult to accept, but we are usually the cause of most of the interruptions that dog us at work. But with the right outlook and close attention to the problem, we can free up a surprising amount of time.

If You Can't Get Your Most Important Tasks Completed at Work

If you ask a few friends to name their greatest frustration at work, you are sure to hear this: "I determine my most important priorities for each day, but I never get to them because of meetings, phone calls, and interruptions."

Without attention, this problem mushrooms into a source of bad stress that cannot easily be chased away. Yet there are many ways to make the situation better:

▶ Set aside "uninterruptible" time blocks each day for your most important duties. You could try getting to work at eight A.M. every day and working behind closed doors until nine. Or go to a vacant conference room or office at midday to tackle your most important tasks. When you utilize private time this way, you are able to deal more calmly with the day's many other activities (meetings, business lunches, interruptions) because they are not in direct conflict with the "core" duties that weigh on your mind.

▶ Don't overburden your daily to-do list with more than two or three items. Jam-packing your daily list doesn't really help you get more work done. It only gives you a chronic feeling of being behind. Instead, keep one list of all your ongoing projects in a place that is separate from your daily to-do list. Then each day, transfer the two or three pressing tasks from that list onto your daily list of projects to complete. If you are not able to accomplish your top priorities on that first day, copy them over to the next day's list. If you still can't get them done on that second day, it's time for some special action. Set aside time in the evening, or early the next morning, to knock them off and clear your to-do list for new items. You can also use commuting time or a Saturday morning in the office.

Many people expect that working extra hours to complete important projects would be "stressful." The opposite is often true. Logging those extra hours may be an unfortunate side effect of the workload most of us carry today, but doing it can actually serve to *reduce* stress.

Take the Sting out of Unpleasant and Stressful Tasks

Perhaps you dread going through your annual job review with your boss. Or you have to meet each month with a demanding customer who makes life impossible for you.

Such workplace stresses can be hard to endure. If you are dealing with several of them in any given week or day, the stress can pile up and become nearly immobilizing. Yet, again, there are ways to reduce the stress they bring.

- ⟩ Tackle your toughest dreaded duties first thing in the day or, in any case, as soon as possible. If a colleague tries to steal credit for one of your ideas in a meeting, go to his office immediately and hash things out. Or if you have to fire someone, do it first thing in the morning instead of worrying about it until the afternoon. By acting sooner rather than later, you remove the harshest part of many stresses: anticipation. The result can be a marked reduction in stress.

- ⟩ Don't "catastrophize" about what you have to do by trying to anticipate all the things that might go wrong. Try to remember that you really cannot predict or control everything that will take place. In many cases, the problem will be resolved more easily than your "catastrophizing" mind is telling you. Even if unexpected problems occur, you will have the expertise to handle them competently.

Improving Stressful Relationships on the Job

So many books have been written on the subject of handing difficult relationships at work, we could not hope to compete with them. Yet here are some basic approaches for making difficult relationships better:

Stick to your own game. Concentrate on doing your own work very capably, without allowing yourself to be drawn into the conflicts or political battles that difficult individuals would like to pull you into. This is the approach recommended by clinical psychologist Dr. Harry Olson in his influential book *The New Way to Compete*. By playing in your own way, you can remain in calm control and actually come out ahead in conflicts because you are playing your own game, not the one that your opponent is trying to draw you into.

▶ Don't play the role of amateur psychologist, especially with the people you supervise. If you manage a chronic latecomer, for example, your goal should not be to understand the underlying reasons why he is late but to explain clearly that you expect an on-time arrival every day. If he or she cannot accomplish that, point out what the next steps will be in company procedures, such as making a formal complaint. Similarly, if you have a troubled relationship with a boss or a peer, don't spend time wondering, "Why does he (or she) behave this way?" or, even worse, "What am I doing wrong in this relationship?" In business, the goal should be to find goal-oriented ways to work with the difficult person, not psychotherapeutic ways to decode his or her difficult behavior. That's beside the point.

In the fray of difficult relationships on the job, it can be hard to remember that letting yourself be drawn into a public conflict can only make you look bad too, as though you and your unstable peer have sunk to the same unprofessional level. Keep to the high road, focus on your work, and you can continue to look more and more capable as the other person behaves in self-sabotaging ways.

Minimizing Conflicts Between Work and Home Life

Again, entire books have been written on this topic. If you are experiencing extreme conflict between working and home life, it would be a good idea to visit a bookstore or library to find a book of advice on the subject. Yet there are focused ways to reduce the sense of conflict. Start by remembering that conflict between work and home usually falls into two distinct areas:

Emotional/psychological stresses that result from being pulled in two directions. ("Trying to please my boss and trying to please my family," as some people have said.)

Actual time conflicts between work and domestic schedules.

The good news is that employers are in great need of good employees today, and therefore more willing than ever to take special steps to keep them on board. It is a better time than ever to speak to your boss or human resources department about the following options:

▶ Telecommuting full- or part-time. This can be a highly attractive option for employers today. If you are able to telecommute entirely from home, the company will save on office space and equipment. If you are lucky enough to have a spouse who receives health coverage and other benefits through his or her job, you can use those factors as negotiating points with your current employer, who can save the cost of benefits by allowing you to telecommute.

▶ Working a "compressed" schedule. You might be able

to work three or four days each week in the office, instead of five, for slightly longer hours.

▶ Become an independent contractor. Today many companies are eager to outsource key functions to external companies, everything from payroll to data entry to Web site design. With gumption, you might be able to create an outside company that your employer uses. If you process medical claims for a medical group, for example, you might start your own company to perform that function from a home office. By making the right presentation of your plan, you might be able to resolve your crippling conflicts between work and home *and* enjoy the autonomy of having your own business.

More Stress-Beating Tactics for Common Workplace Problems

To reduce your chronic bad stress on the job, pick and choose from the following pinpoint tactics:

If you get too many e-mails, answer them in batches during three half-hour "blitzes" every day: when you arrive at work, after lunch, and at the end of the day. Respond to messages only when it is absolutely necessary, since the more messages you send, the more responses you get.

If you are frustrated by phone tag, include "anticipatory" information in the messages you leave. Example: "Chris, we missed again. If you were calling to see if I can attend the meeting next Friday, I'll be there."

If people drop into your office and take up too much of your time, stand up when they arrive and remain standing during the conversation. The sense of urgency will keep discussions shorter. And whenever you can, hold meetings in *other* people's offices since it is easier to get up and leave than to usher visitors from your office.

If you lose time going to meetings you don't need to attend, ask if you can be put on the distribution list for minutes. Or ask whether you can attend only the sessions where your specific input is needed.

If you supervise people who argue, don't intervene more than twice. Simply state that you expect cooperation at once and an end to the skirmishing.

If you are just plain overworked, tactfully begin to say no to new assignments. You can even say to your boss, "I am also handling assignments A, B, and C as top priorities. Can you tell me where this new project fits in, and which I should handle first?" In this way, you reduce the number of assignments on your to-do list without seeming uncooperative.

If you deal with one annoying activity through the day, such as handling repetitive customer complaints on the phone, find a way to deal with them on the first call, not the second or the third. One approach is to present a list of the problems you are encountering to your supervisor ("I'm hearing these same three complaints repeatedly . . .") and ask for clear instructions on just what you can do to resolve them on the spot.

If callers take up too much of your time chatting, cut them off politely with a statement like "Glad to hear from you, but I'm in a crunch, so what can I do for you?"

18

WHEN TO SEEK PROFESSIONAL HELP FOR YOUR STRESS

When should you admit that your personal resources are inadequate to manage the stress in your life? When it is time to seek the help of a psychotherapist or other professional to manage distress, anxiety, or depression?

First, avoid engaging in self-blame. After all, speaking with a psychologist or other professional represents just one more technique to find help for stress, similar to all the others you have encountered in this book. According to Kenneth D. Cole, Ph.D., clinical associate professor of psychology at the University of Southern California, who is an expert in the area of stress:

> To blame ourselves or to try to "fix" ourselves in the context of overriding anxieties about work, relationships, or other distress can be pure folly. In many cases anxiety, depression, and general "distress" are important signal emotions that we so commonly dismiss or disregard as we try to keep on going . . . If you are feeling anxiety or depression that doesn't seem to go away after several weeks, and you can't identify clear reasons for these symptoms of distress, that is when you could consider consulting a mental health professional such as a clinical psychologist, psychiatrist, or psychiatric social worker.

According to Dr. Cole, treatments for anxiety and depressive disorders have demonstrated some of best outcomes of all mental health interventions. In other words, chances are good that short-term therapy will help you obtain relief from anxieties or depression you can't manage on your own.

Following are stress-related disorders for which Dr. Cole suggests professional intervention.

Habitual Worrying: Generalized Anxiety Disorder

Chronic anxiety, habitual worrying, and the inability to relax are signs of generalized anxiety disorder, one of the most common of all psychiatric disorders in America today.

Even though generalized anxiety disorder usually responds well to short-term psychological intervention, few sufferers seek treatment. For them, anxiety has become so routine, they don't see it as aberrant. Neither do they appreciate how much the problem erodes their enjoyment of life. However, there are reliable clinical protocols for dealing with this troubling problem, especially cognitive-behavioral techniques that should require a course of between five and twenty sessions with a psychologist.

"If some enterprising therapist offers you only long-term treatment consisting of several sessions a week over a period of years, seek another opinion," Dr. Cole advises. He also states that some sufferers of generalized anxiety disorder enjoy positive benefits from nonaddictive medications such as BuSpar (buspirone) and in some cases Neurontin (gabapentin). However, regular use of drugs such as Ativan or Valium, once commonly used to treat "free-floating" or "existential" anxiety, should be avoided. "While very appropriate for episodic use or during a period of acute stress, the regular use of these drugs leads to tolerance when more of the drug is needed to feel the same positive effects, and possible addiction."

Extreme Shyness: Social Anxiety Disorder or Social Phobia

What's the difference between social phobia and simple shyness? To decide, mental health professionals weigh the degree of functional impairment caused by the sufferer's problems. If you're worried about shyness, it's wise to remember that some degree of social anxiety is quite normal. For example, it has been widely reported that death is the second greatest fear among Americans. The first is public speaking. In another example, golfers typically say they feel the greatest inhibition about their skills when teeing off on the first hole; a location where they can typically be observed by other golfers lingering around the clubhouse.

In contrast, someone suffering from a true social phobia feels highly conflicted in all social settings. He or she often longs for social connectedness and is highly sensitive to any signs of rejection. Consequently, many sufferers restrict their activities and engage in activities only where it is obvious that they are wanted and valued. Feeling uncomfortable in social situations, they harbor themselves away in an attempt to avoid the pain of rejection.

Shyness, even *intense* shyness, responds well to professional help. Cognitive-behavioral therapies have been developed expressly for the treatment of such disorders, along with a number of newer medications with indications for these problems.

Specific Phobias

Specific phobias, once called simple phobias, are fears tied to specific situations or events. The sufferer might sense acute stress when anticipating or experiencing events such as:

- exposure to certain animals or insects
- natural events such as storms, earthquakes, or heights
- enclosed spaces such as elevators
- receiving injections or other medical procedures
- driving, flying, taking other modes of public transportation, or going through tunnels

In extreme cases, the sufferer can even faint. Often these symptoms develop in childhood and sometimes they are shared by members of the immediate family.

When is it advisable to seek professional help for such phobias? According to Dr. Cole, professional intervention is advisable when fears get in the way of your functioning or keep you from living a happy and productive life. Typically they are amenable to simple cognitive-behavioral therapies that might include a gradual exposure to the feared object or situation.

There is another option too. In some cases, it may be quite practical to get on with your life by simply avoiding the anxiety-inducing situations or events. After all, staying away from snakes if they cause you anxiety will not cause any erosion in your well-being! According to Dr. Cole, it's also wise to set aside the "Hollywood psychology" of years past that promulgated the notion that superficial phobias were signs of more serious pathologies lurking below the surface. "There is no sound evidence for this rather romantic notion," he observes.

Obsessions and Compulsions

Simple obsessions are recurrent thoughts, images, or impulses that the sufferer has a difficult time controlling. Compulsions are their physical counterpart, actions such as repeated hand washing (along with a Jerry Seinfeld-like fear of dirt and germs), extreme orderliness and ordering, excessive checking to make sure an appliance is turned off, or the repeating of words or phrases silently to oneself.

A person who is experiencing obsessions or compulsions feels driven to perform these mental or physical rituals, often according to some rigid system of rules, in order to lessen building tension and anxiety. Thinking about or performing the act temporarily reduces anxiety until it mounts once again.

Dr. Cole advises that although these problems appear dire, they usually respond well to short-term cognitive-behavioral psychotherapy, now often coupled with the use of medications that were initially used as antidepressants.

When is it vital to seek help for these stresses? Again, the issue is one of decreased function. Often people don't realize how severely simple obsessive/compulsive problems can impact on happiness. If you are experiencing the stresses that arise from these obsessive patterns, short-term therapy should provide relief.

Acute Stress Disorder and Posttraumatic Stress Disorder

The problem of anxiety received a great deal of attention in the months following the terrorist attacks that took place on September 11, 2001. And with good reason. Persons who have experienced, witnessed, or been confronted with an event that involved actual or threatened death, injury, or harm to physical integrity are ripe for developing an acute stress disorder, which by definition resolves within about four weeks or posttraumatic stress disorder (PTSD), which can linger far longer. PTSD is common among war veterans, but victims of auto accidents, physical assaults, and sexual trauma may experience it also.

According to Dr. Cole, there is much controversy over whether critical incident debriefing, when counselors are flown in to trauma zones to help the witnesses and survivors, does anything to prevent the onset of acute and chronic posttraumatic stress disorders. In order for feelings of stress to dissipate, some people want and need to talk about the event over time.

Others choose to be left alone with their thoughts and feelings, a preference that should be respected by members of the health-care professions. "Carelessly prescribing the same 'correct' treatment is not good clinical practice and is effrontery to people suffering the ravages of a horrible event," Dr. Cole observes.

If an acute stress disorder does not resolve within several months after a traumatic event, you might be well advised to seek professional help. Some indications that you should do so might include still being hounded by dreams and/or daytime flashbacks of the event and being reminded of the event by smells or weather conditions, bringing on symptoms of stress.

Short-term therapies and counseling can again help. If your sleep is disrupted, a physician or a psychiatrist can prescribe medications on a temporary basis to help you get needed, restful sleep. Certain antidepressant medications have also been shown to be useful medications for PTSD as well. In fact, Zoloft now has a specific indication for PTSD. But your doctor may prescribe one of a range of newer antidepressants for the "off-label" use for PTSD, when PTSD is not listed on the medication's label or in accompanying pamphlets and has been shown to help the condition.

Chronic Depression: Dysthymia or Dysthymic Disorder

These terms refer to a low-level chronic depression lasting for a year or more in children and over two years in adulthood. Many of us can feel anxiety and/or depression for several months after a significant loss, whether the death of a loved one, the loss of a job, or more enigmatic feelings of losing a sense of prestige or importance in the world.

Bereavement is an allied problem. Uncomplicated bereavement typically resolves within a year, and thereafter any lingering feelings of guilt surround only the issues regarding the loss.

For example, a grown child may feel guilty that he or she didn't visit his ill mother enough or had neglected to tell her how important she was.

Various stressful life events may cause anxiety and depression, and these feelings usually dissipate over the course of several months. But if you're a person who has felt continuously depressed for years and have accompanying symptoms like chronic difficulties maintaining sleep, eating too much or not having an appetite, low energy, little interest in sex (whatever your age), poor concentration, guilt and self-recrimination about many aspects of your life, or poor self-esteem, you may be among the millions of Americans who suffer from dysthymic disorder.

For generations, people tolerated these kind of feelings and symptoms, even hiding them from public view. At last, many people are giving up their lives of "quiet desperation" and are reaching out for support. Psychotherapy is often more exploratory for a condition like dysthymia, but cognitive-behavioral, interpersonal, psychodynamic, and other psychotherapy approaches may be effective with this problem. In fact, in the last dozen years or so, the same antidepressants described above are being utilized for this condition, especially because the burden of side effects is typically much less with these agents than the older medications.

Life is too short to go through it suffering in silence. With the development of specific, scientifically tested psychotherapies and new medications, it is tragic to let your life slip away for the fear of "exposure" as someone who is depressed.

Major Depression

If your depression is so severe that it drastically impacts your day-to-day functioning (and if you may be thinking of death or suicide), then you have met the criteria for what is now called major depression. This condition is further classified into unipolar and bipolar depression, the latter being the downswings of what was once called manic-depression and now is referred to bipolar disorder.

Severe biologically driven unipolar depressions and all bipolar disorders have a strong familial link. Often, extended family histories are replete with depression or withdrawn women, alcoholic men, very "checkered" life histories full of indiscretions, and even suicides.

Major depression is a very painful problem and needs prompt and aggressive psychological and psychiatric attention. The new antidepressant medications mentioned above are used for this difficulty, often coupled with psychotherapy. In very severe or refractory cases, electroconvulsant therapy is still used, but only after a demonstrated lack of response to many medications now available.

The treatment of bipolar mood disorder, marked not by daily fluctuations in mood but by protracted mood changes over months, is outside of the scope of this book and is treated with medications other than antidepressants, such as lithium carbonate and now often Depakote.

Other Concerns

If you are experiencing intense anxiety or abject depression for the first time in your life, see your primary care physician, who can rule out any of many medical conditions that cause anxiety and depression as part of their presentation. Also, alcohol abuse and both prescription and illicit drugs can cause depressive symptoms.

Talk about such problems with your physician. For example, chronic alcohol dependence can cause a smoldering depression, and even the casual use of cocaine can cause severe dysphoria after use.

Taking Away the
Stigma from Medications

As stated earlier in this chapter, an important first step toward finding relief from unmanageable stress is to reject the idea that we should be blamed for seeking professional help. A similar observation can be made about taking medications for certain disorders that we are finding it hard to otherwise control.

"When you take a medication for a common psychological malady," Dr. Cole observes, "there is the implicit notion that you're fundamentally defective, and you need to take this given agent as remedy to make you whole again."

While not all therapeutic approaches to treating the anxieties and disorders described in this chapter will include the use of prescription medication, some may. It is a decision that only you can make, based on your own comfort level with taking medications coupled with the best advice of a qualified professional. However, avoiding all medications in the belief that you should be able to solve all your problems without them might cut you off from a source of relief that has become accepted medical practice in the last decade. Many new psychiatric medications are being developed by pharmaceutical companies and then approved by the FDA once their clinical efficacy and safety have been established.

Today, taking appropriate medications under professional supervision does not mean you are seriously mentally ill or unable to respond to other therapies. It may simply mean you are taking advantage of the most effective and latest therapies to help bring your problems under control.

A Final Word:
On Becoming a Stress Master

This book is now finished. Does that mean our work is done? No, not at all, for a simple reason: As long as you and I live, every day will bring us new and unexpected stresses.

You and I can choose to react blindly to all those new stresses. We can jump straight into fight or flight mode at the slightest provocation. Or, using the skills we've learned in this book, we can commit to a lifelong process of making the most of the good stresses that come our way and minimizing the damage done to us by the bad. The result can be a life that is not only lived capably but extraordinarily well.

All it takes is bravery, flexibility, good humor, and a certain keen eagerness to take action in the face of life's challenges instead of sitting passively by.

It has been a joy to share the explorations of *Good Stress, Bad Stress* with you. I hope that for you the journey has just begun.

APPENDIX:
YOUR PERSONAL
STRESS INVENTORY

What stresses you?

When you respond to that question, you will probably point to only a few stressful areas in your life. You will probably respond with just one answer, or possibly two.

"My job's hectic pace."

"Debt."

"My relationship with my boss."

"My dealings with my former spouse."

"My diabetes."

"Conflicts with my kids."

Of course, those are perfectly valid areas for you to feel stress in your life. However, because the purpose of this book is to help you deal effectively with all the stresses in your life, we need to dig deeper. The Personal Stress Inventory that follows is designed to do just that.

Set aside about forty-five minutes, without interruption, and check the boxes that apply. If a question does not apply to you, simply skip it and move on to the next.

Move along quickly and have fun. If you find yourself wavering about which response to check, go with the answer that was your first impulse.

> Note: Because many of the following questions are highly personal in nature, you might want to photocopy your Personal Stress Inventory and keep it in a private place instead of completing it in the book, where family members or friends might see your responses.

Global/National Issues

1. Concerns about national security
- ❑ highly stressful ❑ stressful ❑ not stressful

2. Worries over family and personal safety
- ❑ highly stressful ❑ stressful ❑ not stressful

3. Concerns about future of America
- ❑ highly stressful ❑ stressful ❑ not stressful

4. Worries about friends/relatives in military or other danger
- ❑ highly stressful ❑ stressful ❑ not stressful

5. Worries about economy
- ❑ highly stressful ❑ stressful ❑ not stressful

6. Current climate and prospects for your business/industry
- ❑ highly stressful ❑ stressful ❑ not stressful

7. Other (please describe):_____

_____

- ❑ highly stressful ❑ stressful ❑ not stressful

Home Life and Routines

8. Shopping for food and household items
- ❑ highly stressful ❑ stressful ❑ not stressful

9. Meal preparation
- ❑ highly stressful ❑ stressful ❑ not stressful

10. Home cleaning
- ❑ highly stressful ❑ stressful ❑ not stressful

11. Yard maintenance
- ❑ highly stressful ❑ stressful ❑ not stressful

12. Religious life
- ❑ highly stressful ❑ stressful ❑ not stressful

13. Patterns of television watching
- ❑ highly stressful ❑ stressful ❑ not stressful

14. Comfort of clothing/footwear
- ❑ highly stressful ❑ stressful ❑ not stressful

15. Issues of home decorating and renovation
    ❑ highly stressful   ❑ stressful   ❑ not stressful

16. Routine driving
    ❑ highly stressful   ❑ stressful   ❑ not stressful

17. Reliability and ease of driving your car
    ❑ highly stressful   ❑ stressful   ❑ not stressful

18. Ease of stocking/retrieving refrigerated items
    ❑ highly stressful   ❑ stressful   ❑ not stressful

19. Laundry/washing routines
    ❑ highly stressful   ❑ stressful   ❑ not stressful

20. Comfort of home heating and air-conditioning
    ❑ highly stressful   ❑ stressful   ❑ not stressful

21. Sleep patterns and routines
    ❑ highly stressful   ❑ stressful   ❑ not stressful

22. Waking up (alarm/clock-radio)
    ❑ highly stressful   ❑ stressful   ❑ not stressful

23. Pets and associated routines
    ❑ highly stressful   ❑ stressful   ❑ not stressful

24. Concern over health of pets
    ❑ highly stressful   ❑ stressful   ❑ not stressful

25. Comfort of your bed
    ❑ highly stressful   ❑ stressful   ❑ not stressful

26. Safety/security of home
    ❑ highly stressful   ❑ stressful   ❑ not stressful

27. Noise level in and around home
    ❑ highly stressful   ❑ stressful   ❑ not stressful

28. Community where you live
    ❑ highly stressful   ❑ stressful   ❑ not stressful

29. Relationships with neighbors
    ❑ highly stressful   ❑ stressful   ❑ not stressful

30. Filing and tracking mail and bills
    ❑ highly stressful   ❑ stressful   ❑ not stressful

31. Phones (unwanted calls, mealtime interruptions, etc.)
    ❑ highly stressful   ❑ stressful   ❑ not stressful

32. Other (please describe)_____

_____

❑ highly stressful ❑ stressful ❑ not stressful

Parenting (complete section if applicable)

33. Children's health issues

❑ highly stressful ❑ stressful ❑ not stressful

34. Schooling

❑ highly stressful ❑ stressful ❑ not stressful

35. Homework routines

❑ highly stressful ❑ stressful ❑ not stressful

36. Cost of education

❑ highly stressful ❑ stressful ❑ not stressful

37. Driving/transport of children

❑ highly stressful ❑ stressful ❑ not stressful

38. Selection/buying of children's clothing

❑ highly stressful ❑ stressful ❑ not stressful

39. Preparation of children's meals

❑ highly stressful ❑ stressful ❑ not stressful

40. Communicating with children

❑ highly stressful ❑ stressful ❑ not stressful

41. Children's spending routines

❑ highly stressful ❑ stressful ❑ not stressful

42. Children's use of alcohol/drugs

❑ highly stressful ❑ stressful ❑ not stressful

43. Children's smoking

❑ highly stressful ❑ stressful ❑ not stressful

44. Children's sexual activity

❑ highly stressful ❑ stressful ❑ not stressful

45. Children's academic work

❑ highly stressful ❑ stressful ❑ not stressful

46. Children's future

❑ highly stressful ❑ stressful ❑ not stressful

47. Children's friends
❑ highly stressful ❑ stressful ❑ not stressful

48. Children's participation in sports
❑ highly stressful ❑ stressful ❑ not stressful

49. Children's driving
❑ highly stressful ❑ stressful ❑ not stressful

50. Children's attitude toward you
❑ highly stressful ❑ stressful ❑ not stressful

51. Worries about school and other violence
❑ highly stressful ❑ stressful ❑ not stressful

52. Children's Internet use
❑ highly stressful ❑ stressful ❑ not stressful

53. Children's choice of music
❑ highly stressful ❑ stressful ❑ not stressful

54. Antisocial/hostile behavior of your children
❑ highly stressful ❑ stressful ❑ not stressful

55. Children's level of help around the house
❑ highly stressful ❑ stressful ❑ not stressful

56. Children's use of television
❑ highly stressful ❑ stressful ❑ not stressful

57. Children's use of phones
❑ highly stressful ❑ stressful ❑ not stressful

58. Mealtime conversations
❑ highly stressful ❑ stressful ❑ not stressful

59. Other (please describe):_____

_____
❑ highly stressful ❑ stressful ❑ not stressful

Marriage/Love Relationships (Note: "Partner" is used to denote spouse or significant other; answer only the questions that pertain to you now.)

60. Fear that you will never meet the right love partner
❑ highly stressful ❑ stressful ❑ not stressful

61. Anxiety about having to end your relationship
❑ highly stressful ❑ stressful ❑ not stressful

62. Concerns that you are involved with the wrong person
❑ highly stressful ❑ stressful ❑ not stressful

63. Quality of communication with partner
❑ highly stressful ❑ stressful ❑ not stressful

64. Your satisfaction in relationship
❑ highly stressful ❑ stressful ❑ not stressful

65. Nature/satisfaction of sexual relationship
❑ highly stressful ❑ stressful ❑ not stressful

66. Concerns about how long relationship will last
❑ highly stressful ❑ stressful ❑ not stressful

67. Concerns about partner's attraction to other people
❑ highly stressful ❑ stressful ❑ not stressful

68. Mealtime conversations
❑ highly stressful ❑ stressful ❑ not stressful

69. Conflicts over child raising
❑ highly stressful ❑ stressful ❑ not stressful

70. Financial discussions and decisions
❑ highly stressful ❑ stressful ❑ not stressful

71. Concerns about spending by spouse or partner
❑ highly stressful ❑ stressful ❑ not stressful

72. Concerns about alcohol use by partner
❑ highly stressful ❑ stressful ❑ not stressful

73. Drug/substance abuse of partner
❑ highly stressful ❑ stressful ❑ not stressful

74. Concerns over health of partner
❑ highly stressful ❑ stressful ❑ not stressful

75. Level of partner's assistance with your health issues
❑ highly stressful ❑ stressful ❑ not stressful

76. Arguing
❑ highly stressful ❑ stressful ❑ not stressful

77. Your partner's driving
❑ highly stressful ❑ stressful ❑ not stressful

78. Your partner's reactions to your driving

❑ highly stressful ❑ stressful ❑ not stressful

79. Compatibility of meal/food preferences

❑ highly stressful ❑ stressful ❑ not stressful

80. Compatibility of health/fitness activities

❑ highly stressful ❑ stressful ❑ not stressful

81. "Bottling up" or avoidance of issues

❑ highly stressful ❑ stressful ❑ not stressful

82. Vacation planning and activities

❑ highly stressful ❑ stressful ❑ not stressful

83. Holiday and entertaining planning

❑ highly stressful ❑ stressful ❑ not stressful

84. Past or current extramarital relationships of you/partner

❑ highly stressful ❑ stressful ❑ not stressful

85. Equitable sharing of domestic duties/routines

❑ highly stressful ❑ stressful ❑ not stressful

86. Equitable sharing of parenting duties

❑ highly stressful ❑ stressful ❑ not stressful

87. Relations with your previous partners/spouses

❑ highly stressful ❑ stressful ❑ not stressful

88. Relations with partner's previous partners/spouses

❑ highly stressful ❑ stressful ❑ not stressful

89. Relationships with partner's children from previous relationships

❑ highly stressful ❑ stressful ❑ not stressful

90. Partner's relationship with your children from previous relationships

❑ highly stressful ❑ stressful ❑ not stressful

91. Compatibility regarding activities/hobbies, etc.

❑ highly stressful ❑ stressful ❑ not stressful

92. Issues concerning maintaining/decorating home

❑ highly stressful ❑ stressful ❑ not stressful

93. Comfort with partner's friends

❑ highly stressful ❑ stressful ❑ not stressful

94. Partner's acceptance of your friends

    ❏ highly stressful   ❏ stressful   ❏ not stressful

95. Relationships with partner's family

    ❏ highly stressful   ❏ stressful   ❏ not stressful

96. Partner's relationship with your family

    ❏ highly stressful   ❏ stressful   ❏ not stressful

97. Compatibility of sleep patterns

    ❏ highly stressful   ❏ stressful   ❏ not stressful

98. Fear of physical confrontation from you/partner

    ❏ highly stressful   ❏ stressful   ❏ not stressful

99. Other (please describe): _____

_____

❏ highly stressful   ❏ stressful   ❏ not stressful

Other Family Relationships (as applicable)

100. Relationship with your mother

    ❏ highly stressful   ❏ stressful   ❏ not stressful

101. Relationship with your father

    ❏ highly stressful   ❏ stressful   ❏ not stressful

102. Relationship with your siblings

    ❏ highly stressful   ❏ stressful   ❏ not stressful

103. Grief/mourning issues for deceased parents/relatives

    ❏ highly stressful   ❏ stressful   ❏ not stressful

104. Ease/planning of family activities at holidays

    ❏ highly stressful   ❏ stressful   ❏ not stressful

105. Problems with healthcare of parents/older relatives

    ❏ highly stressful   ❏ stressful   ❏ not stressful

106. Expenses associated with parents/older relatives

    ❏ highly stressful   ❏ stressful   ❏ not stressful

107. Other (please describe): _____

_____

    ❏ highly stressful   ❏ stressful   ❏ not stressful

Finances

108. Preparation and filing of taxes
    ❏ highly stressful   ❏ stressful   ❏ not stressful

109. Maintenance/filing of financial records
    ❏ highly stressful   ❏ stressful   ❏ not stressful

110. Concerns for amount of money saved
    ❏ highly stressful   ❏ stressful   ❏ not stressful

111. Debt
    ❏ highly stressful   ❏ stressful   ❏ not stressful

112. Concerns over debts of partner/spouse
    ❏ highly stressful   ❏ stressful   ❏ not stressful

113. Cost of medical/health care and medications
    ❏ highly stressful   ❏ stressful   ❏ not stressful

114. Financial planning for retirement
    ❏ highly stressful   ❏ stressful   ❏ not stressful

115. Investments [ ] highly stressful
    ❏ highly stressful   ❏ stressful   ❏ not stressful

116. Relationship with broker/financial consultant
    ❏ highly stressful   ❏ stressful   ❏ not stressful

117. Insurance costs and coverage
    ❏ highly stressful   ❏ stressful   ❏ not stressful

118. Ability to pay monthly bills
    ❏ highly stressful   ❏ stressful   ❏ not stressful

119. Ability to pay for heating
    ❏ highly stressful   ❏ stressful   ❏ not stressful

120. Ability to pay for food
    ❏ highly stressful   ❏ stressful   ❏ not stressful

121. Ability to pay taxes
    ❏ highly stressful   ❏ stressful   ❏ not stressful

122. Cost of housing
    ❏ highly stressful   ❏ stressful   ❏ not stressful

123. Saving/costs for children's education
    ❏ highly stressful   ❏ stressful   ❏ not stressful

124. Ease of using your bank and its services

❑ highly stressful ❑ stressful ❑ not stressful

125. Cost of maintaining home

❑ highly stressful ❑ stressful ❑ not stressful

126. Cost of owning/maintaining car

❑ highly stressful ❑ stressful ❑ not stressful

127. Decisions about purchases of items for the home

❑ highly stressful ❑ stressful ❑ not stressful

128. Other (please describe): _____

❑ highly stressful ❑ stressful ❑ not stressful

Job and Career

129. Ability to manage workload

❑ highly stressful ❑ stressful ❑ not stressful

130. Hours spent on the job

❑ highly stressful ❑ stressful ❑ not stressful

131. Overall pace of job

❑ highly stressful ❑ stressful ❑ not stressful

132. Business travel [ ] highly stressful

❑ highly stressful ❑ stressful ❑ not stressful

133. Ease of using required computers/technology

❑ highly stressful ❑ stressful ❑ not stressful

134. Issues of sexual and other harassment

❑ highly stressful ❑ stressful ❑ not stressful

135. Commute to and from work

❑ highly stressful ❑ stressful ❑ not stressful

136. Comfort of office/workplace

❑ highly stressful ❑ stressful ❑ not stressful

137. Repetitive nature of work

❑ highly stressful ❑ stressful ❑ not stressful

138. Physical danger of work

❑ highly stressful ❑ stressful ❑ not stressful

139. Seasonal "ups and downs" of work

❑ highly stressful ❑ stressful ❑ not stressful

140. Confidence in ability to perform job well
      ❏ highly stressful   ❏ stressful   ❏ not stressful

141. Job setting (indoors, outside, office ventilation, lighting, etc.)
      ❏ highly stressful   ❏ stressful   ❏ not stressful

142. Relationship with your boss or supervisor
      ❏ highly stressful   ❏ stressful   ❏ not stressful

143. Relationship with your colleagues and coworkers
      ❏ highly stressful   ❏ stressful   ❏ not stressful

144. Relationships with company leaders
      ❏ highly stressful   ❏ stressful   ❏ not stressful

145. Relationships with people who report to you
      ❏ highly stressful   ❏ stressful   ❏ not stressful

146. Relationships with important vendors
      ❏ highly stressful   ❏ stressful   ❏ not stressful

147. Lack of support staff
      ❏ highly stressful   ❏ stressful   ❏ not stressful

148. Meetings
      ❏ highly stressful   ❏ stressful   ❏ not stressful

149. Deadlines
      ❏ highly stressful   ❏ stressful   ❏ not stressful

150. Budget
      ❏ highly stressful   ❏ stressful   ❏ not stressful

151. Interruptions
      ❏ highly stressful   ❏ stressful   ❏ not stressful

152. Phone tag
      ❏ highly stressful   ❏ stressful   ❏ not stressful

153. E-mail [ ] highly stressful
      ❏ highly stressful   ❏ stressful   ❏ not stressful

154. Clutter and paper flow
      ❏ highly stressful   ❏ stressful   ❏ not stressful

155. Opportunities for advancement
      ❏ highly stressful   ❏ stressful   ❏ not stressful

156. Uncertainty about long-range career options
      ❏ highly stressful   ❏ stressful   ❏ not stressful

157. Overall career satisfaction

❏ highly stressful ❏ stressful ❏ not stressful

158. Comfort with company values and activities

❏ highly stressful ❏ stressful ❏ not stressful

159. Feelings about job security

❏ highly stressful ❏ stressful ❏ not stressful

160. Confidence about ability to find a job if laid off

❏ highly stressful ❏ stressful ❏ not stressful

161. Concerns about layoffs/downsizing/acquisitions, etc.

❏ highly stressful ❏ stressful ❏ not stressful

162. Concerns about workplace violence

❏ highly stressful ❏ stressful ❏ not stressful

163. Delegating to your staff

❏ highly stressful ❏ stressful ❏ not stressful

164. Comfort with company culture and norms

❏ highly stressful ❏ stressful ❏ not stressful

165. Conflicts about honesty/integrity of your job

❏ highly stressful ❏ stressful ❏ not stressful

166. Giving/getting performance reviews

❏ highly stressful ❏ stressful ❏ not stressful

167. Firing people/making layoffs

❏ highly stressful ❏ stressful ❏ not stressful

168. Makine speeches/presentations

❏ highly stressful ❏ stressful ❏ not stressful

169. Office politics

❏ highly stressful ❏ stressful ❏ not stressful

170. Workplace meal routines

❏ highly stressful ❏ stressful ❏ not stressful

171. Comfort with job-related parties, social events

❏ highly stressful ❏ stressful ❏ not stressful

172. Other (please describe):_____

_____

❏ highly stressful ❏ stressful ❏ not stressful

Health

173. Concerns about aging
      ❑ highly stressful   ❑ stressful   ❑ not stressful
174. Personal weight issues
      ❑ highly stressful   ❑ stressful   ❑ not stressful
175. Eyesight
      ❑ highly stressful   ❑ stressful   ❑ not stressful
176. Issues of healthy diet and eating habits
      ❑ highly stressful   ❑ stressful   ❑ not stressful
177. Smoking
      ❑ highly stressful   ❑ stressful   ❑ not stressful
178. Alcohol
      ❑ highly stressful   ❑ stressful   ❑ not stressful
179. Issues of drug use/abuse/dependence
      ❑ highly stressful   ❑ stressful   ❑ not stressful
180. Self-care of chronic conditions and illnesses
      ❑ highly stressful   ❑ stressful   ❑ not stressful
181. Relationship with physicians and care providers
      ❑ highly stressful   ❑ stressful   ❑ not stressful
182. Costs of medications and care
      ❑ highly stressful   ❑ stressful   ❑ not stressful
183. Satisfaction with healthcare plan
      ❑ highly stressful   ❑ stressful   ❑ not stressful
184. Concerns about exercise or lack of exercise
      ❑ highly stressful   ❑ stressful   ❑ not stressful
185. Concerns about anxiety or depression
      ❑ highly stressful   ❑ stressful   ❑ not stressful
186. Worries about sudden or unexpected illnesses
      ❑ highly stressful   ❑ stressful   ❑ not stressful
187. Costs of medications and care
      ❑ highly stressful   ❑ stressful   ❑ not stressful
188. Suicidal or violent thoughts
      ❑ highly stressful   ❑ stressful   ❑ not stressful

189. Other (please describe): _____

       ❑ highly stressful   ❑ stressful   ❑ not stressful

Overriding Personal Issues

190. Dissatisfaction because life is not what you expected

       ❑ highly stressful   ❑ stressful   ❑ not stressful

191. Concerns about how stressed you are

       ❑ highly stressful   ❑ stressful   ❑ not stressful

192. Disappointments with your accomplishments

       ❑ highly stressful   ❑ stressful   ❑ not stressful

193. Issues of self-worth and self-esteem

       ❑ highly stressful   ❑ stressful   ❑ not stressful

194. Worries about your future

       ❑ highly stressful   ❑ stressful   ❑ not stressful

195. Belief that life is/has not been worthwhile

       ❑ highly stressful   ❑ stressful   ❑ not stressful

196. Relationships with other people

       ❑ highly stressful   ❑ stressful   ❑ not stressful

197. Loneliness

       ❑ highly stressful   ❑ stressful   ❑ not stressful

198. Fear of the future

       ❑ highly stressful   ❑ stressful   ❑ not stressful

199. Satisfaction with religion/spiritual issues

       ❑ highly stressful   ❑ stressful   ❑ not stressful

200. Other (please describe): _____

_____

       ❑ highly stressful   ❑ stressful   ❑ not stressful

Commentary

Congratulations! You have now completed the Personal Stress Inventory and have a much more complete picture of where stress is at work in your life.

We also have a surprise for you. Almost all people, when completing this self-test, find that they are checking the middle "stressful" box most of the time. About midway through the inventory, they start to wonder "Is anything wrong with me? Am I really this stressed in all of these areas?"

The inventory was designed that way, because the areas we are really concerned about are the two that fall on either side of that middle box: the "highly stressful" and "not stressful" responses.

The "highly stressful" responses point out stressful problems that need your first attention and processing using the techniques explained in this book. We will explore:

- whether these acute stresses might be areas of good stress in disguise
- if they are really bad stresses, whether they have the potential to be changed to good
- if they are really bad stresses, and likely to remain that way, how their negative impact can be reduced

There is also a lot to be learned from your "not stressful" responses. In some cases, they are inconsequential. If your children's drug use is not stressful to you because your children don't use drugs, for example, then why should the problem stress you?

But in other cases, your "not stressful" responses contain valuable lessons about areas where you are already dealing effectively with issues that could easily be causing you a great deal of stress and concern. Perhaps you and your spouse deal with financial issues without stress or your career is comfortably stable and secure. Those are no small accomplishments and perhaps you can learn lessons from them that can be used to improve pockets of negative stress in your life.

Before you move on to the chapters in this book, take one final step. Under each of the categories listed below, write the numbers of the inventory items ("34, 121," etc.) where you checked "highly stressful." They will serve as a personal blueprint for the stresses you will process using the techniques in *Good Stress, Bad Stress*.

Global/National Issues_____

Home Life and Routines_____

Parenting_____

Marriage/Love Relationships_____

Other Family Relationships_____

Finances_____

Job and Career_____

Health_____

Overriding Personal Issues_____

ACKNOWLEDGMENTS

Heartfelt thanks to the many wonderful people who lent their support, ideas, and enthusiasm to this book.

Thanks to my wife, Fran, and my daughter, Olivia, for everything they did, every day, to support me at every stage of this project.

Thanks to Gareth Esersky, the kind of agent writers dream about, for her steady stream of enthusiasm and ideas.

Thanks to Matthew Lore of Marlowe & Company for his visionary leadership over this project from first day to last.

Thanks to Dr. Ken Cole, psychologist and lifetime friend, for his ideas, support, and careful review of the manuscript.

Thanks to Nina Frost, Ken Ruge, and Dick Shoup, therapists and career counselors whose great compassion for people set the tone for my writing.

Thanks to my brother Dave, the real writer in the family, for helping me keep my head on straight during the entire process.

Thanks to Larry Levenson, who told me that clarity is what makes a writer good.

Thanks to third-grader Leah Hirsch and to her mom, Donna, who stopped by the bench where I sometimes write to see how the book was coming along.

Finally, special thanks to the the hardworking people I have met and interviewed through my years as a journalist and writer. Little did you or I know that the things you taught me would turn up in this book about stress.

ABOUT THE AUTHOR

During his twenty-year career as a journalist and author, Barry Lenson has interviewed many people engaged in high-stress, high-risk professions, including high-wire walker Philippe Petit, lion tamer Gunther Gebel-Williams, opera singer Marilyn Horne, as well as CEOs, baseball and basketball coaches, athletes, secretaries, orchestra conductors, and assembly-line workers. He has been editor of *Executive Strategies, Working Smart, The Organized Executive,* and other newsletters and has recently been named director of publications for the American Executive League. His books include *Simple Steps: 10 Things You Can Do to Create an Exceptional Life* (with Dr. Arthur Caliandro) and *Take Control of Your Life* (with Dr. Richard Shoup). Barry Lenson earned degrees from McGill University and Yale. He lives with his family in Millburn, New Jersey.